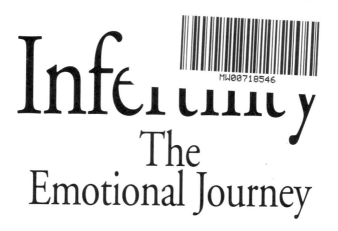

Infertility
The
Emotional Journey

Michelle Fryer Hanson

DEACONESS PRESS
Minneapolis

Published by Deaconess Press (a service of Fairview Riverside Medical Center, a division of Fairview Hospital and Healthcare Services), 2450 Riverside Avenue South, Minneapolis, MN 55454

Library of Congress Cataloging-in-Publication Data

Fryer Hanson, Michelle.
    Infertility : the emotional journey / Michelle Fryer Hanson.
        p.   cm.
    ISBN 0-925190-74-8 (trade paper) : $10.95 ($12.95 Can.)
    1. Childlessness--United States--Psychological aspects.
    2. Infertility--United States--Psychological Aspects.   I. Title.
HQ536.F78   1994
304.6'32--dc20   94-5929
                                                                      CIP

First printing: March, 1994

Printed in the United States of America
98 97 96 95 94   7 6 5 4 3 2 1

Cover design by Tabor Harlow
Cover illustration by Jodie Winger

Publisher's Note: Deaconess Press publishes books and other materials related to the subjects of physical health, mental health, and chemical dependency. Its publications, including *Infertility: The Emotional Journey,* do not necessarily reflect the philosophy of Fairview Hospital and Healthcare Services or their treatment programs.

*This book is dedicated to the two most important
people in my life: To my husband, Duane, who was always at
my side and has supported me through the journey of infertility.
To my beautiful daughter, Mary, who has renewed
my faith and filled the hollow in my soul.*

TABLE OF CONTENTS

ACKNOWLEDGMENTS

Just as it isn't possible to survive infertility without help, it wasn't possible to write about infertility without support and assistance.

I would like to thank all the people who shared their stories for this book. It was difficult for many of them to talk about what they had gone through, but they all found the strength because they felt sharing their stories might help others in dealing with infertility.

Special thanks to Dr. Michael Fiegen and the caring and professional staffs of the OB/GYN Clinic and Sioux Valley Hospital for providing excellent medical care during my struggles with infertility and pregnancy.

And finally, thanks to my sister Kim, who encouraged me to write this book and who tenaciously kept track of my progress.

INTRODUCTION

I am broken
like a malfunctioning computer
with wires plugged into nowhere
Information inputted
Information outputted
No consolidation occurs

I am broken
like a doll with no head
The neck has been broken, unsalvageable
With both pieces together,
a joy to play with
When broken, it's discarded, useless
It sits on the shelf

I am broken
like a wild animal who has been beaten,
the spunk and life taken away
The animal remains whole
but the life is gone
It feels nothing

I am broken
like an infertile woman
All parts are there
But they refuse to make
a functioning whole
No joy or love can be produced
No miracle performed
Life's most precious gift denied
because I am broken

This poem is dedicated to the fifteen to twenty percent of the couples in the United States who are infertile. I wrote it when I was at one of my own low points with infertility. I know each and every infertile couple will hit these lows; it is this book's purpose to acknowledge the great emotional pain and grief that are part of infertility.

As my husband and I struggled with infertility and the whole gamut of emotions that it entailed, I looked for ways to cope. Most of the time, I ran up against a wall. I found no books like this one to help me see that we were not the only ones suffering, and friends and family did not seem to understand. Society does not readily help the infertile couple. Most people do not understand the isolation and desperation that come with infertility. And what people do not understand, they tend to avoid. In our case, my husband and I looked to one another for comfort. There was solace there, but it took a long time to find. We also looked to God, but in the depths of our desperation and grief, we thought He was not there.

This book consists of the stories of individuals' struggles with infertility. It collects case study accounts of how real people have faced their infertility problems. It has no easy answers or magical cures; it is a heartfelt exploration of seven infertile couples' journeys. Each situation in the book is different, just as every reader of the book has their own individual story. But there are common threads that run through all cases of infertility. These are threads we each must cling to in order to truly realize that we are not alone. This book has been written from the individual's perspective. It is by no means a step-by-step medical guide to infertility. The medical procedures detailed are the individuals' recollections of treatments.

No matter what the infertility diagnosis is, or how long one suffers through infertility, the process is intrusive. Infertile couples have to struggle to live normal lives. There is so much emotional debris that gets in the way of everyday living that its existence must be acknowledged.

In most cases of infertility, the marital relationship is deeply affected. Research studies clearly indicate that one of the largest problems infertile couples face is conflict over the differences in the way each person grieves and deals with infertility. Men are more likely to have an optimistic outlook and be less emotional than women. They tend to deal with the situation by taking one day at a time or by trying to forget the problem.

Women, on the other hand, tend to be more emotional and grieve openly. Whenever these differences cause problems, open communication between both partners is essential so they may learn appropriate ways to grieve together.

Relationships with close friends and family are also affected. The infertile couple tends to become more isolated from others as the partners move further through their infertility treatment. The reason is that most people do not understand what the infertile couple is facing. They assume that a pregnancy will occur eventually or utter insensitive statements without even realizing it. The couple's feelings of grief and sorrow are minimized by assumptions that a pregnancy will eventually happen. While the couple feels anguish, friends and family are angered or confused by the couple's seemingly pessimistic attitude.

Money also becomes an ever-looming problem for an infertile couple. Most health insurance companies do not cover many of the costs of infertility treatments. In order for a couple to conceive, they may spend hundreds of dollars a month. For infertile couples, staying at their place of employment can be vital to keep the insurance in effect.

Time becomes rigidly controlled in the infertile couple's lives. A great deal of time is spent at the doctor's office. The couple may never know with certainty when a test will be scheduled, when ovulation will take place, or even when they can make love. Time is no longer the couple's; infertility dictates how they may use it. Life always feels like it is on hold— it is rarely spontaneous and seems to happen in spurts. Vacations and spur-of-the moment leisure activities are virtually eliminated from a couple's lives. Life is broken into two-week segments: the first two weeks anticipating ovulation and conception, the last two weeks wondering if a pregnancy occurred. Infertility is also intrusive when the couple has difficulty enjoying themselves in certain situations. My husband and I hated hearing about or seeing couples who were pregnant or had new babies. Infertility made a once pleasant situation unbearably painful, so we avoided it whenever possible.

With infertility there also come unanticipated emotional triggers which are different for each couple. An emotional trigger is anything that makes the couple feel smothered by their infertility. For us, emotional triggers included holidays, the sight of new parents holding their babies, the smell of baby shampoo, the feel of soft baby blankets, and insensitive statements. To make matters worse, a couple never knows what might act as a trigger until they encounter it.

Infertility makes the natural process of trying to conceive clinical and unnatural. All sorts of tests and procedures intrude, and the infertile couple never gets a break from the condition. It is always there. The pain and sorrow of infertility are always at work on the couple.

Infertility is unlike other situations that require one to grieve. Unlike the death of a loved one, there is never a sense of finality to the grief. It is a repeating cycle that becomes more intense with the passage of time.

An infertile couple is on an emotional roller coaster. There are too many feelings to deal with effectively. The cycle of emotions includes hope, anxiety, fear, anger, sadness and grief, and it starts anew with each new menstrual cycle.

Infertility makes a couple constantly reexamine their beliefs. Infertility treatments are intrusive and can be very demeaning; couples need to decide if the treatments fit in with their already-existing beliefs. As they go through the process of trying to conceive and give birth, they must constantly restructure old philosophical and religious beliefs to fit their current situation.

To my husband and me, perhaps the most difficult part of infertility was that it made us feel like we were all alone. We felt there were very few people out there who wanted to understand our problems, and that those who did were unable to. Like the other couples in this book, we lived through infertility. As you read these stories, I hope you will find solace in the words. You are not alone, and there more and more of us each year who understand your devastation.

There are many paths one can take on the journey of infertility, all leading to different destinations. You are the one who will ultimately decide on which path you choose. For some couples, the path leads to the resolution of a child-free lifestyle. Others may pursue infertility treatments or adoption. If you choose to pursue a baby and do not give up your dream, we believe you will get your baby. The baby may or may not be your biological child, but it is our firm belief that it is the one God intended you to love and care for.

1

MICHELLE AND DUANE'S STORY

From Michelle's diary, January, 1991:

> *I finally came to the realization today that I can't afford surgery this month. This is my last month on Clomid and I know I am not pregnant. Because our financial situation is so precarious at this point, I am not sure when I will be able to have the surgery.*
>
> *I feel so bad. I wish someone could fix me. Make me normal like everyone else. I have blamed God a lot lately. I know I shouldn't, but I want to. Why is He letting this happen to us? Are we such bad people that we don't deserve a baby?*
>
> *One of my college students told me that. I don't know if she knew about my situation or not—some people know, and things get around. She said that the reason there is infertility is because God knows certain people are not worthy of children. I know she is wrong. There are thousands of children who are beaten and killed by their parents every year. Parents who would harm their most precious gift are certainly not worthy, yet they have babies.*
>
> *I have been compiling a list of idiotic, insensitive phrases I have heard since we have begun this process:*
>
> - *"Don't try so hard. You'll get pregnant in no time."*
> - *"You can always adopt!" (Duane and I just called the state social services department and they told us to call back in a year and we might be able to get on the waiting list then. Private adoption would be a choice, but is very expensive. This is something that is not possible for us at this time.)*

- *"Children aren't all that they are cracked up to be."*
- *"Did you hear so and so is pregnant?" or, "Did you hear so and so just had a baby?"*
- *"Well, you really haven't been trying very long. Be patient and it will happen."*

I have heard all these and more. They tear my heart out, especially when the words come from a close friend or family member. People who haven't suffered through infertility have no idea of how much their careless words hurt us. We are not only hurt by infertility, but by society's ignorance.

The diary I kept during our long struggle with infertility was one of the ways I coped with the endless frustration of hopes raised and dashed in regular two-week cycles, with well-meaning but thoughtless friends and relatives, and with the constant fear that things would never work out, that we would never have our baby. Even now, years later, it tears me apart to read these entries, to dredge up the pain I'd hoped I'd put behind me. But the tears and anger I committed to paper during those terrible times kept me sane enough and strong enough to go on, to continue the struggle with infertility, to be a survivor against adversity.

As I write this, my husband and I have been married for eight years. When we were first wed, we wanted children, but not right away. We felt we needed to find out about each other before we brought a new life into the world. So we planned on having a child when I finished my bachelor's and master's degrees.

About three years into our marriage, however, I started having baby pangs. I saw other couples with their babies and thought Duane and I would make great parents, but Duane reasoned that we should wait until I finished school and we could more easily afford a child; still, I had a difficult time waiting. I had been halfway into completing my master's degree when I started to pester Duane about babies.

During this time we were invited to a friend's wedding in Iowa, where my husband served as the best man. At the reception we had a wonderful time, drinking too much and enjoying each other's company immensely. Just before the bride and groom's first dance, we were informed that the entire wedding party would participate in the next dance. This was dreadful news, because Duane and I could not dance to save our lives. However, since it was important to the newlyweds, we acquiesced.

The bride and groom danced to Anne Murray's song, "Can I Have This Dance for the Rest of My Life?" It was very romantic. By the time it was our turn, I felt so happy and relaxed that I could have danced anywhere. The music was slow and compelling, and as I danced close to my husband I whispered in his ear, "Is it time for our baby yet?" He looked at me for a long time, smiled, and then said, "Ask me tomorrow." By the look in his eye and the tone of his voice I knew he would say yes.

The next morning we met the rest of the wedding party for breakfast. As we sat jammed into a small booth, I asked my husband, "So what's your answer?" He looked at me, squeezed my hand, and said, "Okay." I was the happiest person alive. I smiled all through breakfast, feeling assured of my impending pregnancy.

The first couple of months that I attempted to conceive were difficult for me. I had been on birth control pills and having regular menstrual cycles. After I stopped taking the pill, I had regular twenty-nine day cycles for two months. Then my cycles became long and irregular. I started seeing symptoms of ovulation and pregnancy in myself when there were none. Each month I truly believed I was pregnant, and I often took pregnancy tests on the thirtieth day of my cycle.

After I would take the tests and find they were negative, I would start crying. Duane reassured me that we had just started the process and that pregnancies don't happen right away for every couple. But after four menstrual cycles, I started worrying about my irregularity. I purchased many books and started learning about my body, female reproduction, and infertility. As I read, I found myself described in the books as a woman likely to have problems with conception. As a teenager I had acne; dark hair on my chest, arms, and toes; irregular cycles; and excessive pain during the first few days of my cycle. Still, since my mother and sister had had the same symptoms, I felt there was nothing abnormal about me. Then my husband found out he was suffering from a prostrate infection. The urologist said there might be a problem with his sperm count, and to check on this if a pregnancy did not occur in six months.

As the months went by without a pregnancy, I decided to start keeping a diary. The turmoil and sadness that surrounded our efforts to conceive overwhelmed me so much that I felt the need to write it down. Each month when my cycle began, I felt like I wanted to die. I kept asking myself, "Why is this so difficult for us? Everybody else can do it. Lots of people do it without even trying!" I was convinced that we were going to need to see a fertility specialist to find out why we were not having any luck becoming pregnant. I remember feeling very anxious and frustrated about our situation. Whenever I asked Duane if we should see a specialist he said I was looking for problems where there were none. My friend, who had struggled with infertility, was telling me I should make an appointment without delay. I didn't know what to do.

I soon discovered that when you are having problems conceiving, babies and pregnant friends are everywhere. My friend Laura stopped by with her newborn, Maria. Laura has been my friend since eighth grade, and had been pregnant twice before. I do not know how those pregnancies ended, but I do know that the decision to keep Maria was a very difficult one for her, as she was single and still in college.

Laura's baby was the most beautiful thing I had ever seen! I watched Laura holding and cuddling the baby and was very jealous. I became more so when I found out that Laura's sister, Sherry, was expecting to deliver a baby within the month. Like Laura, she was young and not married. It made me so sad—so many women get pregnant and don't want to be. I wanted to be, and all I had was sorrow.

Still, it was so much fun to watch Maria stare at my husband, Duane. He was so gentle with her; I knew he would make a good father. I wished and prayed I could give him that opportunity, but at times a pregnancy seemed impossible to me. And all around me were people with babies, with easy, often unexpected pregnancies, with all the joy and happiness that seemed so far away to me.

I had told my friends and family that we were finally going to start a family. Each month people would ask me if I was pregnant yet. At first, it was exciting to have everyone so interested in our plans. After a few months, however, I cringed as soon as the words came out of their mouths.

After a few months of failing to conceive, I started taking my basal body temperature to help pinpoint ovulation. To do this I had to take my temperature the same time every morning and chart the results. When my temperature dropped it was an indication of my most fertile time;

after ovulation, my temperature would rise a few tenths of a degree. The day the menstrual cycle would begin, the temperature would drop again. Each month I would grieve when my temperature went down.

As the months passed I became more and more upset to find out I was still not pregnant. When I started to bleed it was as if I were experiencing a death—not of a person, but a death of hope and optimism. My reaction bothered my husband. He felt I should not be so pessimistic and should instead look towards the future. But after nine months of grieving and many heated discussions, Duane agreed we should contact a fertility specialist. My friend who had a history of infertility problems had suggested I see her doctor, a reproductive endocrinologist, so I made an appointment to see him.

Three months later we went to the appointment. It was nerve-wracking for us. We were unsure of what would be done and what the doctor would find out. But we were also excited—we felt we were finally moving ahead and dealing with the problem.

The doctor did a pelvic examination on me, and then called my husband and I into his office. He said I had endometriosis and possibly enlarged ovaries. He explained that endometriosis was caused when blood from the menstrual cycle backs up into the body and makes deposits on the surrounding organs. These deposits turn into scar tissue, which makes it harder for conception to occur.

He also explained that I had a hormonal imbalance which was causing me to experience long and irregular menstrual cycles. The doctor wanted to do a laproscopic procedure, which entailed a scope being inserted into my navel so he could could examine my reproductive organs. Although I was anxious about the surgery, I also looked forward to it. To me, the surgery signified hope. The most irritating part of our session, however, was that he addressed Duane. He was talking about me, about my condition, as if I wasn't there. When I asked questions, he looked at Duane as he answered. His treatment of women seemed to be a relic from the stone age, but because I had been told that he was an excellent doctor and I believed he could help us have a baby, I agreed to let him perform the surgery.

The laproscopic surgery was a same-day procedure; I entered the hospital early in the morning and was in and out of surgery in a couple of hours. It was a strange but interesting experience. One minute I was awake and feeling fine on the operating table, and the next I awoke in the recovery room, feeling quite a bit of pain. I remember slowly becoming aware of a sharp burning in my stomach, and complained to the nurse about the pain.

Duane was so worried for me. He was there when I woke up, helping me swim out of my groggy haze, and when I complained about the pain, he pestered the nurses to get medication for me. Although it sometimes felt like we were so far apart on our feelings about infertility, I knew I could not get through these difficult times without him.

After I recovered from the anesthesia, the doctor came in to talk to us. He had found that my tubes were free of obstruction, my ovaries were enlarged, and that I had endometriosis. During the procedure, he had cauterized most of the scar tissue that was the endometriosis, but he also thought I had a cyst on my ovary that might make ovulation difficult. He gave me the option of four months on the fertility drug, Clomid, or surgery to remove the cyst. Unlike the laproscopic procedure, this surgery would require a three-day hospital stay and a ten-day at-home recovery.

Still groggy and in pain, but feeling some hope, I was sent home with a bottle of prescription-strength Motrin and the advice to rest and recover for a few days.

I had been led to believe that this procedure meant that I would be able to get around on my own, as long as I took it easy. We left the hospital in the afternoon and even though I was still groggy, I was quite hungry. I asked my husband to stop at a fast food restaurant for lunch. By the time I made it from the car to the booth, I felt like I was going to pass out. I was dizzy, shaking, and was nauseous. It took about a week before I felt fully recovered from the procedure.

As I was recovering from the laproscopic surgery, Duane and I discussed our options. The surgery would be more expensive, but would give us a better chance of conceiving. The Clomid was both the more conservative and far less expensive option. We chose the Clomid treatment, reasoning that if it wasn't successful, we still had the option of surgery.

Clomid is a mild fertility drug that is taken days five through nine of the menstrual cycle to induce ovulation to occur at around day fourteen of the cycle. The doctor had indicated that it was also necessary at this point for Duane to have a sperm count done. It was Duane's first direct involvement with infertility treatments and he was a bit embarrassed and uneasy about what was required. He had to ejaculate into a jar and deliver the jar to the medical lab. But as time and treatments went on, both Duane and I learned to do whatever was needed, and although we overcame embarrassment, some uneasiness always remained.

After Duane's test we waited impatiently for the outcome, not knowing which way our treatment was going to go—further tests and possible surgery for Duane, which would delay my treatment, or Clomid for me. The results of the sperm count were adequate—Duane's sperm count and motility were fine—so I began to take Clomid.

The first month on Clomid the doctor asked us to come in for a post-coital (PK) test. This test enabled him to determine if my cervical mucus was thin enough for the sperm to make the journey into the uterus. We had intercourse two hours before seeing the doctor, and he removed a sample of mucus from my vagina to determine its consistency. He informed me that since my husband's sperm count and motility were good, my mucus was thin enough to facilitate sperm movement.

We went home feeling that we were finally on the way to having a baby. We were more than ready to stop the awful grieving process we had been experiencing. But during the next three cycles I realized there was a thickening of the mucus. After four cycles on Clomid I did not get pregnant. The doctor had recommended surgery as the next step if Clomid was not effective, and had not discussed any other options. In February of 1991, I wrote the following entry in my diary:

> I found out today I'm not pregnant. I could barely climb out of bed. I don't want to do anything. I want to sit under a rock until I find out I can finally have my baby. Duane feels bad, but I feel worse. I can't seem to quit crying. Duane says I'm too pessimistic and that I have not even given us a fair chance. He yelled at me to quit crying. I can't blame him because I know that he is hurting too. He just doesn't understand this deep fear of mine. The fear that I will never have my own baby. That we will be alone for the rest of our lives.
>
> I have no one to talk to. Not my family or my friends. I've tried, but

they don't seem to understand. Duane suggested a counselor, but I don't think I can go to one. I need to talk to someone who has gone through this. Someone who knows my pain and grief without any explanation.

I told my family and friends of our plans for a baby, and every month they used to ask if I was pregnant. Now I'm embarrassed to talk to them. I know they don't understand why I don't feel happy anymore.

At least most people have stopped asking me if I'm pregnant. They must all know the answer is no.

Due to the expenses of graduate school, our financial situation was less than secure, so we decided to wait a few months before proceeding with the surgery. I had purchased supplemental insurance through a professional organization I had joined, which would help with the expenses, but it would not cover "preexisting" conditions until nine months after the policy began.

The decision to wait was incredibly difficult for both my husband and I to make. We cried a lot and started feeling more depressed than ever. While Duane was sad and hurting too, he couldn't understand the depth of my pain. In my diary I wrote:

I am chastised for grieving. Duane sees me as a manipulator and accuses me of making these feelings up to make him feel bad. He will never know how empty I feel. No one will. The pain of the first day of my cycle hurts, but it is nothing compared to the pain of feeling hollow, unable to ever conceive a child. Every cramp reminds me of my failure. I can't afford the second surgery, so I will have to postpone it. This kills me. It puts off what small chance I have for a pregnancy by months or years. When will the tears stop? When will the grieving and loss vanish? When will my longing be answered?

During this time we checked into the possibility of adoption. Both Duane and I come from families familiar with adoption: I have a cousin and Duane has twin nieces who are adopted. Duane made calls to state and church-sponsored adoption agencies. The response was the same at all of them: the waiting lists are two years long and are closed. There are far more people who want to adopt a baby than there are babies available.

They each suggested we call back in a year, and perhaps the waiting lists would have opened. A check into private adoption revealed that this option was very expensive and could also be very complicated. We decided to continue to try to get pregnant, and, if necessary, explore adoption further at a later time.

Before we looked into adoption, we had no idea that it would be difficult to adopt a baby. I had always heard that adoptions took awhile, but the babies were there. We were shocked to find out that it was almost impossible to adopt a white child under two years of age through a public agency. When I told people this, they almost invariably asked, "If you want a child so bad, why don't you adopt an older child or one with special needs?" Every time I heard this I felt guilty. I wanted to raise a beautiful, healthy baby. Was that wrong? Was I being selfish? The fact that I wanted a baby became one more reason for my self-esteem to plummet even further.

While we waited for the chance at the second surgery, I was again overwhelmed by the number of babies and pregnant friends all around us. Sherry's sister Laura was pregnant again, and my mother's friend Emily was about to deliver. Phone calls and letters from friends often meant news of pregnancies, and these friends quite rightly wanted us to share their joy. But it was too difficult; we could not be happy, and our friends didn't deserve to be brought down by our pain.

So we found ourselves not writing letters, not answering the phone, not answering the doorbell. Other people's joy was too much to deal with, and we retreated into an isolation that allowed us to be alone with our fears and grief.

I recall watching the movie *Immediate Family* on television at about this time. The main character, played by Glenn Close, was dealing with infertility, and calling people to cheer her up. An acquaintance on the phone asked her, "So, are you pregnant yet?" The question. The horrible, hateful question that every infertile couple dreads hearing. As I watched the scene play out before my eyes, I felt she was me. Her experience was mine and I wept as I watched.

For me, the most affecting scene from the movie was when the main character's husband, played by James Woods, went to a football game with some of his friends. As they walked by an alley in the stadium he saw a father with his little boy. They were hugging and laughing and the camera showed the husband's reaction. In that moment I could see all of Duane, and all my pain and hopes. It hurt to watch that scene, because I felt the pain just as strongly as the character in the movie. I thought that maybe if everyone saw that movie, they might understand our situation a little more. Shortly after that I wrote the following entries in my diary:

> *I remember praying to God after I got my first menstrual cycle. I asked Him to take away my period and that if He did I wouldn't care if I couldn't get pregnant. Well, I still have my period, but no baby. Not exactly fair play. Now I pray that God will grant me the chance to have and raise a baby… I have asked, and asked, and asked. I wonder if anyone listens? Does God?*

> *My friend Andrea has had a very difficult time with her fertility as well. She has three beautiful children, but she has lost many pregnancies. I talked with her today. She told me that it's okay to be mad and that it is okay to hurt, but I should never believe that my pain is God's will. She believes we were given free will and because of that, there is evil in the world. God does not want the evil to happen, He does not want the pain and sorrow to exist, but it must exist if people are to have free will. It really helps me to talk to her. She doesn't have all the answers, but she shares my pain. I never have to explain or apologize for the feelings I have. I think people need someone to share their crises with. I think God is helping me through this crisis through my friendship with Andrea. She is a great comfort to me.*

> *Events suggest—no, scream out—that I write in my journal. Last week we got a letter from our good friends. They announced in their letter that they were six months pregnant. They were married in May 1989, which was the time when Duane and I decided to start our family. I was crushed by the news. Duane went to see them when they came to Brookings to visit, but I declined to go. It would hurt too much.*

> *Tonight Andrea came into my office and said she was not a good friend because of something she had done. I thought she was going to tell me something about work. Instead, she told me she was pregnant.*

The news was the shock of the century to me. It is painful, but ironic, and I am okay with it. I pray to God that she will be able to keep that baby. She has lost so many before. She deserves this one. If God cannot give me my baby now, I hope He will keep her baby safe.

Once our supplemental insurance coverage took effect, I contacted our fertility specialist's office again to schedule the surgery he had recommended. However, I was told that the doctor had discontinued his practice because of poor health. The nurse on the phone told me that my case had been referred to another doctor, and that I could continue my care with him.

Hearing this news was one more blow to my already fragile state of mind. Now we were faced with the prospect of starting over from scratch with another doctor. Not only would we have to go through another infertility workup, we would have to establish a rapport with a new doctor. Well-meaning but clumsy family and friends had made us feel that we were the only people in the world with fertility problems; to approach yet another stranger and confess our apparent inadequacies as baby makers seemed to be a monumental effort for both of us.

We made an appointment to see the doctor the following month. Our first impression was not a good one. He was two hours late for our appointment, and then he apologized to us because he said he had not yet read our medical file. I grew more and more agitated as he talked. I remember thinking, *We're asking for the most important type of help, and our doctor hasn't even read our file!* But since we had waited so long, we let the doctor go ahead with the fertility workup. He informed me that I did not have a cyst on my ovary—surgery was unnecessary—and recommended another prescription of Clomid.

I was confused and apprehensive about this. This new doctor's recommendations were so at odds with those of my previous doctor that I was not sure I could believe him, so I started asking questions. Months of reading every book and article on infertility I could find had given me the ability to discuss all aspects of the proposed treatment. To my surprise, the doctor answered all my questions thoroughly and gently. I began to realize that although he had made a bad first impression, he was a competent, reassuring, caring physician. And best of all, he talked directly to me. He treated me as an informed, intelligent woman who had a right to be a partner in her own medical decisions.

We had been on Clomid only a short time with our previous doctor, and were willing to give it another chance. For the next four menstrual cycles I was on Clomid. I would come in for an appointment after the start of each new cycle. During this time the doctor would check my ovaries for cysts. Around the fourteenth day of my cycle I would come in for a PK test. This doctor found that my mucus was too thick to facilitate sperm movement, so he gave me estrogen tablets, Doxacycline, and Robitussin to help thin the mucus. After four cycles, he decided that none of the medication was working.

During these months we had gone back to living life in two-week segments—two weeks of hope, only to be crushed by the beginning of my next cycle, which set up a tailspin into two weeks of despair. Then we began the whole process over again. Clomid made my cycle regular, but I also experienced elevated mood swings, tremendous hot flashes, and, just to add to the misery of failing to become pregnant, more painful periods than usual. The misery of the drugs and the failure to become pregnant had me doubting whether all of it was worthwhile. I wrote this entry in my diary:

> *I dream of being pregnant almost every night. I beg God in my dreams to let me have a baby. I wake up in the morning feeling exhausted and drained... Maybe I would be happier if I just accepted the fact that Duane and I will be childless.*

Duane and I became so desperate that we began to grasp at straws. In order to cope with infertility, we became incredibly superstitious. If I wore an outfit to the doctor and received bad news, I made sure never to wear that outfit to another appointment. We went to lunch before each of our appointments, and when a pregnancy did not result, we made sure never to order the same menu items again. Irrational thoughts would enter my head, and I would think that if I did or said something it would mean a pregnancy would result. I remember thinking at one point, *If you don't turn around in a circle three times, you won't get pregnant.* It immediately struck me as an idiotic idea, but I felt compelled to turn around in a circle three times. Logic and common sense were often tossed aside in the hope that magical thoughts and actions would help.

After four unsuccessful months on Clomid, the doctor then told us the next step was artificial insemination using my husband's sperm. We quickly agreed to the procedure. Although the method was unnatural, it at least gave us a chance of producing a pregnancy.

I started using an ovulation kit to try and figure out the day of ovulation. A woman starts taking the test anywhere from day ten to day thirteen. The test is a stick that is placed in the urine stream for a short time. The kit tells you if you are about to ovulate. When I took the test on a Sunday and got a positive result, I called Monday morning for an appointment to be artificially inseminated.

The process consisted of Duane ejaculating into a jar and taking the sample to the lab. At the lab the sperm underwent a process known as "washing." The technicians filtered out the semen and impurities to produce the best possible sample. The washing process, we were told, would take about two hours. At the end of two hours we called the clinic, and they told us to come in immediately.

When we arrived, anxious and excited, they told us our regular doctor was not on call. They then showed us to another doctor's office. In solemn tones he told us that for some reason Duane's sperm count was not adequate to perform an insemination. He advised us to get another sperm count taken to ascertain what the problem was.

This news would have been difficult enough to handle if it had been delivered by our regular doctor, but hearing it from this stranger was simply too much. I felt like we were spinning helplessly out of control. We left the office feeling extremely let down. Once again, there were barriers in our path. Another problem. Another delay. Another month without a pregnancy.

Duane had another sperm count done, and it turned out to be adequate. While we were waiting for the results, however, we had discussed the possibility of using a donor, and all that decision would entail. Duane was receptive to the idea of a donor if that was what would be necessary for us to get pregnant. (Certainly donor sperm, adoption, and other options are all complicated issues, and each couple has to come to their own conclusions as to what is right for them.) When Duane's sperm count came out okay, we set the idea of a donor aside but kept it available as an option.

The next month, December, I realized I was taking longer to ovulate than normal. The doctor did an ultrasound to determine how far along the egg was in development. He gave me a shot of Pregnyl, which speeds ovulation. Two days later I ovulated, and we waited anxiously to hear if Duane's sample was normal. It was, and I was inseminated.

The process was much easier than I had imagined. The sperm sample was in a syringe and was injected directly into my uterus. I then lay on the examining table for twenty minutes to give the sperm the best chance to make its way through the uterus. I left the office feeling optimistic—after all, it was Friday the thirteenth. We had been having such incredibly bad luck that I figured maybe our luck would change on a day known for bad luck.

Our fortunes did not improve, however, and in January the doctor changed my prescription for Clomid from fifty milligrams to one hundred milligrams to make sure ovulation occurred on time. When I ovulated we drove down to the clinic for the insemination. We were full of hope, but when I was in the examining room I heard a lab technician talking to my doctor. My heart sunk as I heard their exchange. Somehow, Duane's sperm motility had inexplicably dropped from fifty percent to ten percent during the washing process.

When I heard them talking I wanted to scream and throw all the books in the room against the wall. How could things like this keep happening? How could our luck keep getting worse? The doctor came in and informed me of the situation. He said he thought we should do the insemination now and do another the next day. I told him I did not think that would be enough time for Duane to build up an adequate count. But I desperately did not want to lose another chance for pregnancy. I inquired about the possibility of using a donor.

My reaction to using donor sperm was positive from the beginning. I felt that sperm was a donation of genetic material only. Essential to make a baby, but irrelevant as far as loving and caring for a child. Duane was ready for us to try donor sperm, too. When we started infertility treatment, he had a more positive outlook and an ability to see the process from a less emotional perspective than I did. But time and disappointment had taken their toll, and he was now as anxious and emotional as

I was. The roller coaster nature of his sperm count, coupled with the inexplicable drop in motility during the washing process had him frustrated. The drop in motility was another complication to an already difficult process.

Duane had made it clear in earlier discussions that he felt there were more important aspects of fatherhood than biology. He said of using donor sperm, "Biologically, our baby will not be mine. But this *will* be our baby, and this baby will be mine in every way that counts. I am looking forward to fatherhood. I am looking forward to helping this baby grow up to be the best person she can be." Time and further tests may have told us why Duane's sperm was so fragile, but neither of us had the emotional strength to deal with further delays. Donor sperm was the obvious answer for us.

Since the day we decided to use a donor, I've been shocked by the number of men I've met who are vehemently opposed to the entire idea. Duane, however, is not surprised by their reaction. He said, "Donor sperm is a very personal decision. I knew some men—and women—would find my decision difficult to understand. I've met men recently who have decided they won't be fathers at all rather than accept a donor.

"I thought about it for quite awhile—Michelle and I had discussed it after our first attempt at artificial insemination, when my sperm seemed nonexistent. There are a lot of issues involved: 'How will this make me feel about the baby? Can I love the baby? How will I feel about myself? Will I be eaten up by feelings of inadequacy? When people learn about the donor, can I handle it? When my baby is old enough to learn about the donor, can I handle it?' One question I didn't consider until later, but which is certainly important, is 'Where does donor sperm place me legally?' I thought each of these questions through, and weighed the need to be a biological father against doing what was necessary for us to have our baby. All in all, it was an easy decision. My only regret is not doing it earlier."

Ordinarily, sperm is ordered and shipped in from a sperm bank in advance. However, since I was already ovulating, we didn't have time to wait. We found out that there were sperm samples available that had been ordered by other couples and never used. If we wanted, we could purchase one of these. Duane and I studied the lists, found an appropriate sample and had the second insemination later that day.

The head nurse told us that if this particular sperm sample did not result in a pregnancy, there were lists of donors we could choose from the next time. The lists were from two different sperm banks. Each donor's height, weight, hair color, eye color, and education were listed. From these Duane and I picked a donor for the next cycle.

Taking this step relaxed us noticeably. Duane was no longer preoccupied with the uncertain nature of his sperm count and motility. Since donor sperm has already been washed and prepared, we were certain we would not waste a valuable ovulation day, and the biological background of our baby was not as important to us as breaking the hold of infertility. Both of us felt that being good parents was more important than being biological parents.

Two weeks later I started bleeding and having cramps. It was not time for my cycle to begin. Lying on the couch helped, and the bleeding stopped soon after it started. I threw up that night and was nauseous the next day. I knew I was pregnant, but I also knew the bleeding was not right. I started to cycle on Tuesday.

I was very upset. I knew I had been pregnant. I knew I had lost my baby. I cried the entire morning I was getting ready for work, convinced I had miscarried.

I work with preschool children in a university lab school, and that day was an orientation session at the preschool. Parents brought in their preschool children, and I knew many would be carrying new babies. I had to be jovial and outgoing as I watched all of the parents with their children. All of these children were beautiful, all of them wondrous gifts from God, and none of them were mine.

When I called my doctor later that day, he confirmed that I had probably miscarried. He told me that many pregnancies end in early miscarriage. After talking with him I was strangely happy, because this was the first ray of hope that I could conceive a child. Even though there was a loss, I was energized with hope.

We kept trying with the donor sperm we had selected, and the March insemination resulted in a pregnancy. It was hard for us to believe that after all this time we were finally pregnant. The first home pregnancy test I took was positive, but be were so excited and so scared I took another. And another. I took four all together—two different brands. They were all positive. I was pregnant at last! We were finally going to have a baby!

I was five weeks along when I miscarried. I had never before felt such overwhelming grief. Duane and I were in shock for over a week.

I had begun spotting on Friday. We were out of town when the spotting began. I had prepared all week for an outreach class I was to teach that weekend in another town. I felt sick on the four-hour trip, but attributed it to exhaustion, apprehension, and the pregnancy itself. We checked into the motel, and being a normal pregnant lady, I rushed into the bathroom.

What happened next seemed like a slow-motion horror movie. As I pulled my white underwear down I saw an intricate pattern of bright red blood. I stared at the underwear for a minute before I started screaming. My deepest fear was becoming a horrific reality. I lay on the bed in the motel room, upset and afraid, while Duane made a series of long-distance telephone calls to my doctor. The type of early miscarriage I was experiencing is common, and none of the medical personnel we talked to was too surprised or alarmed.

On Saturday we drove over two hundred miles to get back home. I cried the entire way. I remember telling Duane I could not believe I was going to miscarry because God would not let that happen to us. Not after all we had gone through to get a pregnancy. I said the words, but I did not believe them.

When we arrived home, we called the hospital, and then drove another fifty miles to get there. Because it was the weekend, our doctor was not available, and we were treated by the doctor on call. This was the doctor who had told us Duane's sperm count was too low, and his compassionate manner had not improved in the succeeding months. While doing an ultrasound, he failed to find a gestational sac, and expressed doubts as to whether we were really pregnant at all. This was an affront to both of us, and Duane, with dry and bitter sarcasm, asked the doctor to put that in writing so we could sue the companies that had made the four pregnancy tests which had confirmed my pregnancy.

Duane's tense sarcasm and the doctor's emotionless demeanor seemed to be on a collision course, and we were glad to leave, to return to our isolated sadness to await the bitter end of our dream. And that end did come, on Monday, with a great deal of blood, and all the tears we had left. We saw our own doctor this time, whose caring and compassion made this terrible and terrifying event as bearable as could be expected. I was miscarrying, and my doctor knew how difficult it was for us.

Before we went to see him, we wrote out a long list of questions for the doctor, because we knew we'd never remember them all otherwise. Why did it happen? Could we have done anything? When can we try again? And more; many, many more. We needed to know why. Why us? Why our baby?

But sometimes there are no answers. We were told there was no definitive explanation for the miscarriage. The doctor said it was probably due to a malformation of the baby; many women suffer the same type of early miscarriage when there is severe genetic damage. It happens so early that most women just think they are suffering a late and extra heavy and uncomfortable period, and never realize that they've had a miscarriage. The doctor then told us that we needed to wait a month before beginning the insemination cycles again.

After the miscarriage, my journal entries were written to the baby I lost. It was my way of coping with loss—to make the baby I hardly knew real:

Dear Lucky,

I miss you so much. We lost you on Friday, April 3rd, when I started spotting. The actual miscarriage was Monday, April 6th. I thought I knew grief. I was wrong—I knew nothing of pain and suffering. I have cried so many tears for you. I am so lonely, so lost.

Although naming you Lucky seems ironic, it is not. God gave me a miracle—you. He could not help that the body you had did not grow. When you died, He took you to heaven. When we get pregnant again, it will be with you. God will not leave us. He will make sure you are with us.

I pray for you every day. Not an hour goes by when I don't think about you. Next time everything will go fine.

Please come home again. We did not lose you forever, just for awhile. I miss you so much I can barely stand it. I know I will get pregnant with you again. I will love you more than you will ever know.

This Saturday you would have been seven weeks old. I miss knowing you are inside me. Nights when I wake up, I have a hard time going back to sleep because I wonder when I will see you again. Going to work is tough too. So many children and babies at the preschool, so many pregnant mothers. I see them and know you should be with me.

You will be with me soon! I know how hard you will fight to come and stay. I hope you never doubt my love, because I would do anything to get you here. There have been many kind people who have helped me through this. All the people at work have been very comforting. Writing notes, sending flowers, saying "I'm sorry." It helps so much. The pain is less when I know others care.

Still, I have also felt great pain. I was going to tell my parents we were pregnant with you on their anniversary, April 10th. I couldn't do that. I know my parents care about me. I know they want to help—they just don't know how. They change the subject instead of letting me vent my grief. I realize intellectually that they probably feel if I don't talk about it I will feel better. That's not true. I need to cry and to scream about my loss. I lost my only baby. I need them to say "We're sorry." But they just don't know what to say, and end up saying nothing.

I hope I never inadvertently hurt you as I have been hurt. I want to be by your side always. We already have an unbreakable bond—you are my baby. Please come home soon. I love you.

I'm so upset with my mom. When I called last night, she asked, "What's wrong with you?" I paused, then said, "Other than losing my baby and feeling miserable every day, nothing." Lucky, I just want her to acknowledge the fact that I lost you and I am grieving. She refuses to ask me about it. When I bring it up, she changes the subject. She is my mother. She is supposed to support me. But all she does is skirt my pain, pretending nothing out of the ordinary has happened. She is always talking about the little girl she babysits. I know this little girl is a large part of her life, but to me it's painful to hear about her. My baby should be that part of her life, not some child she is babysitting. I'm afraid I'll never get the support I need from her.

A co-worker just came into my office to talk with me. She insinuated that I should not have gotten excited over you so soon. She said mis-

carriages are so common that I shouldn't have been excited until later in the pregnancy. How could she say that? I waited three long, painful years for you. I loved you before you were conceived. I enjoyed every minute I was pregnant with you. I hate it when people judge me or try to make me feel guilty for wanting you. I loved you! I still do. I will never let anyone take that from me.

As my diary entries reflect, dealing with the aftermath of the miscarriage was difficult. To be so close to our dream and have it plucked from our hands was devastating. I had a hard time not hating myself because my wretched body expelled my precious baby. I felt responsible for my baby's death and I briefly considered suicide as a way to stop hurting. I prayed to God instead. I asked Him to make me strong enough to continue living.

Each event that went by was marked in my mind by how far along the pregnancy would have been—Duane's birthday was twelve weeks; our anniversary, fourteen weeks. The waiting until we could try again, until we could get our baby back, seemed endless.

During the wait I had the opportunity to take a better job. It was a teaching position at a larger university, at a higher academic rank and with more pay. The city was one in which Duane would have an easy time finding suitable work in his profession as well. It was very tempting, and under other circumstances I would certainly have taken it. But it was in another state, too far away to continue seeing our present doctor. We discussed it, agonized over it, and finally I turned it down. Our first priority was having our baby. Starting over again and perhaps jeopardizing our chances was just too frightening.

Finally, we went back on the insemination schedule, and it almost looked as though it would work right away. I felt like I was having pregnancy symptoms, and my period didn't show up when expected. About the time I had decided to take a pregnancy test, I began to spot. I went ahead and took a test anyway—it was negative.

I had been teaching a weekend adult class, and in my hopeful joy, the night before I had told the women in my class that I was pregnant. I truly thought I was, and all weekend they told me how happy they were for me. I couldn't bear to tell them that I was wrong, that I had let my dream override harsher reality. I continued to write to Lucky in my diary:

How can I love you and want you so much? I don't know your sex, your hair color, your eye color, or your personality. I had you with me for such a short amount of time that I didn't get to know the physical you. But I do love you. I can't wait until we are together again. I pray that you will be conceived with this insemination. If you love us the way we love you, please come home. I know you can with God's help.

Today is our lucky day. We went to Sioux Falls for insemination. Please come home today. Before going to the clinic I bought a lucky pair of socks for you and found a lucky penny on the sidewalk. After the insemination I held on to the sock and penny and chanted, "Lucky sperm and lucky egg, make a lucky baby." The actual procedure took longer than usual, and it hurt! I have a good feeling about this time. I think you had an excellent chance to be conceived. We love you, Lucky.

I got pregnant again during the June insemination. Duane and I were ecstatic, but each day we worried over this new baby. After the first miscarriage we dreaded every twinge of pain, every sensation. Everything went well until we were six weeks along. We had a terrible scare.

It began late one night, when I started having pains on my right side. I went to work the next morning only to come home a couple of hours later because I felt ill. The pains on my right side went away when I lay down, but Duane came home worried, and we decided I should go see the doctor.

Before we could call for an appointment, I went to the bathroom, and as I pulled down my pants I discovered they were saturated with blood. I started yelling and became hysterical. Without pulling my pants up I ran to Duane. He held me in his arms as the blood cascaded down my legs.

I became hoarse from screaming. I finally calmed down enough to pull up my pants and let Duane help me to the car. We rushed to the doctor, certain of the worst. I can't begin to explain what was going through our heads; outwardly we were both strangely calm, perhaps numbed by the shock of yet another disaster, or perhaps we had finally both given in to hopeless resignation.

When we got to the doctor's office we were taken to the ultrasound room. Duane sat beside me, holding my hand. Both of us cried, certain that we had miscarried again, that this baby, too, was lost. Then, as the ultrasound technician recorded the scan of my uterus, she said some of the sweetest words Duane and I had ever heard: "Gestational sac noted. Cardiac activity noted." And there our baby was on the ultrasound. A pulsing point of light. Still there, still alive. The most beautiful sight we could imagine: our tiny, living baby. We cried harder, and dared, once again, to hope.

My corpeus luteum had burst, resulting in the gush of blood. The corpeus luteum cyst provides progesterone to the body to keep the pregnancy viable for the first ten weeks of the pregnancy. I was given a shot of progesterone and my level was monitored thereafter. I was also advised to avoid all strenuous activity and get extra rest for the next four weeks. It was a serious situation, a threat of miscarriage, but if we could get through the next few weeks, we would put this crisis behind us.

It is never easy for me to be totally inactive, not even on doctor's orders, but I did it. I didn't go to work, I didn't work at home; I rested in bed or on the couch, with books and television and boredom, but I did rest. Duane did the laundry, dishes, vacuuming and overall household maintenance. He had always done most of the cooking. We knew that if we could get past two months, the immediate danger would be lessened. For several weeks, we walked on eggshells. Duane said, "Each time my phone rang at work, I was scared it would be Michelle with bad news. I've never been one to pray, but I prayed every day for the baby, and for Michelle. I was a bundle of nerves all through the pregnancy, but I couldn't show Michelle. She needed me to be calm, to be a pillar of support."

We breathed a great sigh of relief when we entered the second trimester of our pregnancy. Every day we had had to fight our fear of miscarrying the baby. While getting to the fourth month did not guarantee a live birth, the odds were now in our favor. In the fifth and sixth months we still had cause to be anxious. The doctor who had done the ultrasound when we miscarried had told me that it appeared I had a heart-shaped uterus instead of the usual pear shape. He explained that this could cause premature labor in the fifth or sixth month. After he told us this, I had consulted my regular doctor. He had said he had noticed the shape on the ultrasound he had done earlier, but felt it was just a shadow. He went on to say that when my original doctor had performed laproscopic surgery he had not indicated any abnormality in the medical records; any such abnormality would have been readily visible to the laproscopic camera. My doctor told me not to worry, that the chance of an abnormally-shaped uterus was slim. Of course, being reassured did not mean we did not worry anyway.

As the pregnancy progressed, we felt and saw our baby move. There are no words to describe my joy and awe as I saw my stomach ripple. Each day the realization came to me anew that I had a living miracle within me. Each day she was getting bigger and stronger.

At seven months, my doctor discovered that my blood pressure was elevating. He advised me to cut back on work, as it looked like I might be developing a condition called toxemia, which is characterized by high blood pressure and excessive water retention. Toxemia can be fatal to both the fetus and mother if not managed properly.

I cut back on my workload and tried to take it easy, resting with my feet elevated at every opportunity. I became increasingly nervous as my blood pressure continued to rise, and my legs and ankles squished with excess water as I walked. I soon started going to see the doctor weekly. Three weeks before my due date, he advised me to stop working and go to complete bed rest. He told me to go to our hometown clinic to have my blood pressure monitored later that week. Just being active enough to have Duane drive me to the clinic was enough to raise my blood pressure to a borderline dangerous level.

Bed rest gave me more time to think, and thus more time to worry. Duane went out and bought a home blood pressure cuff and took my readings every four hours. As long as I was resting the readings were just within the limits my doctor had mentioned. When the readings became higher that weekend, we phoned the on-call doctors twice. They told us that the readings did not yet warrant induction of labor, but that my doctor would probably want to induce labor when I went in for my weekly appointment the following Wednesday. We must have been an irritation to the on-call doctors that weekend, but we needed all the reassurance we could get. We had come too far, gone through too much to take any chances now. We were worried about our baby, and weren't about to apologize to anybody about it.

We packed a suitcase on Wednesday and drove to the clinic. My doctor told me that my blood pressure had gone down a bit and that I had lost six pounds of fluid due to the bed rest. He gave me the choice of another week of bed rest or having labor induced that day. He warned me that the baby had not yet dropped into position and that there was only a fifty percent chance that I would be able to deliver vaginally. Duane and I had talked it over earlier, and we both were certain of the route we wanted to take. There was no way either of us could get through another week of worrying; it was time to have our baby, by whatever means was necessary.

My doctor explained how he was going to go about inducing labor. He planned to give me two doses of Prostoglandin gel, eight hours apart, and ten hours later he would start a Pitocin drip. I was admitted to the hospital and my doctor administered the first dose of gel, the purpose of which is to soften the cervix and spur contractions. The day passed with few contractions, and at 8:00 p.m. the on-call doctor came in to administer the second dose. The on-call doctor turned out to be the same one who had given me the ultrasound when I miscarried, and while everything we had heard indicated that he was very good at his job, his cool demeanor had never endeared him to either Duane or myself. In addition, he always seemed to be the doctor on-call when things had gone wrong for us—just coincidence, but our experiences had left us superstitious and easily bothered, so he was not the doctor we had hoped to see.

As always, he was cool and perfunctory. He applied the gel and left. The next morning we learned that immediately upon leaving my room, he had called my doctor and told him that he might as well save me a lot of pain and useless effort by performing a caesarean first thing in the morning. In this doctor's judgment there was absolutely no chance I would deliver vaginally.

Had I known what that doctor was thinking at the time, I probably would have agreed with him. The first dose of gel had had little apparent effect, and in the hours immediately following the second dose, not much more seemed to happen. As Duane sat by my bedside, we discussed the likelihood of a caesarean delivery, and prepared ourselves for this eventuality.

At 3:00 a.m. I awoke to steady contractions. Duane was sleeping fitfully in the chair beside my bed, and I woke him and asked him to time the contractions. They were about eight minutes apart. We were both glad something was finally happening, but tried not to let ourselves get too excited, so we didn't call the nurse immediately. When she came in to check on me later, she admonished us for not letting her know about the contractions right away. We didn't care—we were too caught up in the moment. At last we were having our baby!

At 6:00 a.m. the Pitocin drip was set up and the contractions quickly became more intense and came closer together. I was surrounded by bulky machines that kept track of my blood pressure and measured the strength of my contractions. Duane wandered around the room nervously, glancing at the readings on the machines and trying, unsuccessfully, to stay out of the way of the nurses. Because of my high blood pressure I had to stay in bed the majority of the time I was in labor.

The doctor came in at 7:00 a.m. and told me I was a fingertip dilated. He discussed pain relief options, and I chose an epidural. An epidural blocks pain from the waist down. (This was an easy choice for me, as I try to avoid pain whenever I can.) I was told the epidural would be administered when I was dilated three centimeters.

There is a window of opportunity for each possible pain reliever in labor; they can't be administered too soon or they will wear off too early, and they can't be administered too late or they can get into the baby's bloodstream. The pain was already significant enough to suit me, and I looked forward to when labor would progress to the point that I could have some pain relief.

As it turned out, my labor progressed so quickly, I didn't get to have the epidural block. When the delivery team realized there would not be time for the block, the backup plan was for a simple narcotic. Again, however, labor was rushing along like an out-of-control freight train, and, after the shot had been prepared, the doctor decided I was too far along, so I didn't get that either. Through the crushing pressure of a contraction I vaguely heard the doctor and nurses talking about how I was not going to get any narcotics. I hoped I had heard wrong, but I didn't dare ask for fear I might panic. I kept up with my breathing and tried to pretend I wasn't in incredible pain. When the doctor told me I could start to push, I was ecstatic. Only a short time until I could hold my baby!

The second stage of labor lasted half an hour. I pushed so hard that I broke blood vessels in both my eyes. (For a few weeks after the birth I looked like a vampire.) The nurse used a mirror to show me the baby's head coming out. She kept encouraging me to keep pushing, and I did.

Moments later the doctor announced that I had a beautiful baby girl. I cried as they laid this most wondrous gift on my chest, then I looked up at Duane standing next to me, and saw that he was crying, too. We laughed as we remembered the on-call doctor's recommendation that I have a caesarean. Not only did I deliver vaginally, but the labor only lasted six hours. We were glad that our doctor had taken a more positive approach and allowed us to make our own choices.

I have always loved sightseeing. Some of my most vivid memories are of beautiful mountains and valleys, of stunning landscapes. All of those sights paled in comparison to the tiny face that looked at me that day. My daughter Mary took my breath away. She was tiny—five pounds, ten ounces, with long fingers and toes and large blue eyes that stared into mine. I felt like I could stare into those eyes forever.

As Duane stood beside me and my mother came into the labor room and saw her grandchild, I finally felt complete. The pain and sorrow of the past several years subsided, to be replaced with incredible joy and peace. In that moment, God had rewarded us for our tribulations. He never stopped loving or caring for us. I will thank him every day of my life for giving us our beautiful little angel.

Since that day I have come to realize that while the birth of our daughter has healed many wounds, the scars of infertility will always be with us. We have learned so many things from living with infertility. We know now that grieving is necessary. We know how important it is to pursue dreams. We know that God will always be with our family.

Our journey of infertility has left us both shaken and empowered. Our lives have been monumentally altered, yet we would not trade our experiences for anything in the world. Through infertility we have become stronger, and we know there are ways to survive crisis. It is our hope that couples who are struggling now as we struggled can find some answers, garner some hope for the future, and triumph against adversity.

2

COLLEEN AND NICOLE'S STORIES

Two Sisters, Two Choices

The following story is about two sisters' struggles with infertility and the different decisions they made. It shows that when more than one sibling is affected by infertility, the situation leads to some very complex family dynamics.

Colleen, the older sister, explained, "Nicole and I never got along until the day I left for college. I think she always wanted to be an only child. But we have become closer now than we ever used to be. There is a connection now that was never there before. On the other hand, infertility distanced us for a time, because we were taking two different routes to the same destination. She chose the doctoring route and I chose the adoption route. The result of this was that we could not follow each other's tracks."

Nicole believes that she and her older sister react very differently to situations in their lives. She said, "I am a big procrastinator, and am not at all aggressive. I try to live life and be happy. If a situation arises at work, the way I deal with it is to hope it goes away. Colleen takes the opposite approach—she hits things head on. It's interesting, though, because when it came to infertility, we changed tactics. Colleen has withdrawn from dealing with her infertility, while I have been searching aggressively for answers. Colleen shuts down when I try to talk to her about infertility treatments. I think there is an emotional line that she will not allow anyone, including herself, to cross yet."

Colleen and Jim met in April, 1986, and married in February of 1987 when Jim was thirty-four and Colleen twenty-six. Colleen remembered,

"Since we knew each other such a short time before we got married, the rumor was that we had to get married. It's kind of funny, because I'm still waiting to have a child; my gestation period would be longer than an elephant's by now.

"We wanted children right away, but we've never been a couple who sits down and plans things. In October of 1987 I started a new job, which required a lot of traveling. Jim's niece was about five years old at the time, and I took her on some of the trips and would practice parenting."

Nicole and Jason were wed in 1988, and from the beginning of their marriage they chose not to use any contraception. They felt that if a pregnancy occurred, they would be ready to start their family. Nicole recalled, "We really weren't in any rush to start a family. We were pretty laid back about the possibility of a pregnancy. If it happened, it happened."

In February of 1988, Colleen went to a family physician to have a routine papsmear done. Colleen explained to the doctor that she had been married for over a year, had not been using contraception, and that she was still not pregnant. Doctor A told her, "Wait until you have been married for about five years before you worry about it." Colleen left wondering if this was truly sage advice or not: "I mentally calculated that if we waited five years, Jim would be thirty-nine, and I would be thirty-one. Although we had never made set plans, we had informally patterned our timeline to have children after my parents'. My parents got married at the same age we did, and I thought that if we waited too long, the pattern would be broken."

In March, Colleen went to Doctor B to be treated for a urinary tract infection. She asked again whether there was a reason to be concerned about a pregnancy not occurring. The doctor told her, "Don't be in such a rush—once you have kids you'll wish you didn't." Colleen said, "At the time I just blew off the idea of a pregnancy. Two doctors basically told me to stop obsessing and not to rush it. In retrospect, I think that by listening to those two physicians we wasted so much time."

A year later, while she was about 400 miles away from her home, traveling for her job, Colleen realized that her period was about two months late. She was ecstatic, and purchased an early pregnancy test thinking that her dreamed-of pregnancy was at last a reality. Her hands were shaking as she picked up the test to read the result. It was negative. A failure. A death of a dream and a blow to her emotional well-being. Colleen said, "I was devastated. I remember the ride home, and it was horrible. It was long and excruciating; time seemed to drag on forever. I drove miles and miles with nothing to think about except for the negative test."

Two weeks later, Colleen still had not started her period. She began to feel hope again, thinking that the last test must have been defective. However, a second test confirmed there was not a pregnancy. Confused, emotional, and tired of hearing the comment, "So when are you going to have some kids?" Colleen made an appointment with a female gynecologist, Doctor C. Colleen explained, "I thought that maybe the men didn't understand me and my desire for a pregnancy. Maybe I needed to see a woman.

"She did a papsmear and a pregnancy test. That test was negative too. She told me I had somatic pregnancy symptoms. She said I wanted so badly to be pregnant that my body was telling me that I was pregnant. Then she gave me a basal body temperature chart, a collection container for a semen sample, and all of those kinds of things. But she acted kind of like I was crazy—I never felt like we connected at all. I never went back.

"We have moved since then, and the semen cup is still in the bathroom drawer. Looking back, I think if she wasn't so insensitive to my needs and did not have such a flippant attitude, I probably would have pursued infertility treatments. At that point I was looking for someone to hold my hand and tell me where I was going. I didn't need someone who acted like I was crazy. Her attitude towards me basically pointed us to adoption."

Largely as a result of that experience, Jim and Colleen decided to pursue adoption through state services in the Fall of 1989. Another factor was that Colleen's mother was a state adoption specialist, and was planing to retire in less than a year. Colleen recalled, "I felt if we were going to adopt, we'd better at least get started with the process before my mom quit."

Jim and Colleen chose adoption through a state agency for a number of reasons. After researching independent adoption sources, Colleen found the cost to be very high. (Another reason for not choosing an independent adoption was that Jim and Colleen knew of a couple that had an infant placed, only to have that infant taken from them when the birth parents changed their minds. Colleen felt that she and Jim could not take that type of heartache.) There was also the fact that her mother, being an adoption specialist for state social services, could potentially offer suggestions in dealing with the system.

In October, Jim and Colleen attended an intensive training workshop for parents who wanted to adopt. In November they worked on their home study. Colleen said, "We found that the waiting lists for babies were closed. For example, in 1992, our state agency only placed two normal, healthy infants. Because we wanted a young child, we decided to pursue adoption of a special needs child. One of the things we needed to do to adopt was fill out a sheet that asked us what kinds of special needs we would accept in a child that we would adopt. I remember my mom just about had a stroke, because I checked just about everything. There were a few things I felt we couldn't handle, like a child with terminal cancer, a child without a limb, or a quadriplegic. Other than those, we were open to just about anything, but I think we were open to everything else because of sheer desperation. I justified it by thinking, *I work in a nursing home, have seen all those conditions, and they don't bother me.* Yet when we had to describe the type of child we wanted, we described a blonde, blue-eyed, normal, healthy child."

Nicole and Jason still had not conceived a baby by January of 1990. Nicole decided to see a gynecologist to seek help in finding an answer to their problem. Jason said, "We knew we'd better see a doctor, because we weren't getting any younger. A lot of our friends were having babies, and it wasn't happening for us."

Nicole went to Doctor C, the same female gynecologist her sister had seen earlier, and explained her and her husband's desire for a baby. Nicole said, "She did a pelvic exam and said everything felt normal. I remember her being very cold, and I felt she didn't take me very seriously. She told me, 'You're young, nothing appears abnormal, so let's not be aggressive at this point.' She basically told me I had lots of time ahead of me. But if you don't know when or even if you will get pregnant, waiting is agonizing. She told me to chart my temperature for six months and come back. I appeared to be ovulating, but she wrote me a prescription for six months of Clomid anyway." Nicole took the fertility drug for two cycles before she quit. Since it appeared that she was ovulating without Clomid, she discontinued the drug. Instead she used ovulation kits to determine when she would ovulate naturally, and timed intercourse.

Nicole was very frustrated. She said, "I wanted a baby so badly, and nothing appeared to be wrong. I would cry and cry at work. I'd have to leave my desk and cry in the bathroom. At the beginning, Jason told me not to cry because he was sure we would get pregnant. But there was just so much missing in my life—being infertile felt like there was a piece of me missing.

"The unknown reason for our infertility was the hardest part. If someone could have told me that in five years I would be pregnant, then I could have been happy. But nobody could do that for me."

As each month passed without a pregnancy, Jason and Nicole felt the strain in their marriage. Jason remembered, "We had a lot of tension between us when we would find out that some of our close friends were expecting. They'd tell us, and we would be happy for them. But then we would come home, not talking to each other, to face our empty house. We had a lot of fights during that time. They weren't about infertility directly, but that was really where they all were centered."

At the same time Jason and Nicole were waiting and hoping for a pregnancy, Colleen and Jim waited to hear about adoption proceedings. In January of 1990, they were informed that their adoption worker had quit. But Colleen's mother, Nancy, kept them informed of where the adoption process was at. Nancy advised Colleen and Jim to revise their home study because she thought their former case worker had done a poor job on it. She made many such comments, but the case study was not redone. Jim and Colleen felt that it was all right the way it was. Colleen remembered, "Right before Mom retired in June, we were visiting a couple who had been in our adoption class. They told us they were just having a little boy placed with them. In our conversation with them we found out that three of the other couples had children placed, while the other couple in our class had never completed their home study. So we were the only ones who had completed the study and hadn't had a child placed—or even been contacted."

January of 1991 was eventful for both sisters. Nicole decided to see another gynecologist, Doctor D, who reviewed Nicole's medical records and did a pelvic exam. He told her he felt no abnormalities, but would like to do a diagnostic laparoscopy to make certain he was not missing anything. In the meantime, he recommended that Nicole go on Clomid for three cycles to see if a pregnancy would occur. He also advised Jason to see a urologist to make sure he was fertile.

Jason had wondered if he indeed was fertile. When he was a few months old he had had a ruptured hernia in a testicle. For all purposes, that testicle was dead. Jason said, "Because my testicle was dead and Nicole appeared okay, we assumed it was my problem. I started feeling very guilty, and then the semen analysis came back showing a high sperm count and good motility. Part of me was very relieved, but part of me was afraid for Nicole."

After the couple found out that Jason was okay, Nicole became very depressed and started to blame herself for their infertility. She said, "It was back on my shoulders. It was hard, because now I felt there was something in me preventing us from having our child. I remember at this point being so low that I really wanted to die. I told Jason that this wasn't the way I thought my life was supposed to turn out. Every month was such a struggle. I was emotionally exhausted and tired of fighting my feelings. The guilt just fed on itself and grew. I felt it would be better for Jason to get on with his life, because I couldn't have his children. I don't remember voicing this concern, but I would pick fights with him and bring up the topic of divorce."

Jason was worried about Nicole's depression and suggested counseling. Nicole remembered, "We talked about going to counseling or attending a support group, but I didn't know about the resources. If you dived into it, that meant making a commitment that infertility was the issue. I felt so abnormal; I think I was afraid to talk to someone else.

"I looked for books to help me cope. I'd buy a book and the cover would say, 'Your Guide to Infertility,' but it never gave me the reasons for unexplained infertility and it certainly offered no concrete ways for me to live through this nightmare. I needed to know if it was normal for me to pick fights with Jason when I got my period. I needed to know if it was normal for me to not feel excited for other people when they told me they were pregnant. These were the issues I was struggling with, and I needed some emotional guidance. There was just nothing readily available on the emotional side of infertility."

While Nicole had been making the decision to see Doctor D, Colleen had called the new adoption worker to ask why there had been no communication since the previous year. Colleen remembered, "Her response was, 'Well, we've changed the process and we don't contact you until we are ready to place.' She seemed irritated that I had the audacity to call and check.

"At the same time, mom was still keeping up with what was going on. She knew that there was a new adoption/foster parent training seminar, and that they weren't placing any children with couples who hadn't gone through this new training process. I felt so helpless. The adoption process is like paddling the wrong way up a raging river—the river is constantly battling you. There was so much time when we weren't in communication with anybody, and then we were told we weren't going to be contacted until they had a child to place with us. I was so angry about their callousness. It was like they just didn't care to give us any information at all.

"Around this time Jim and I heard that there was a sibling group of six children, all boys, all under eight. We talked seriously about adopting them. My mom nearly had a stroke when she heard about it. She told me that I couldn't do my own laundry, let alone six other people's. She talked us out of it. I think at times she would have talked us out of adoption altogether if we would have been open to that."

In March, Jim and Colleen attended a fundraising breakfast. While there they met a couple who were foster parents in their community. The woman turned out to be one of the instructors of the new adoption/foster parent training seminar, and encouraged Colleen and Jim to attend the classes. The couple had brought their foster child with them—a four-month-old boy who had been with them since December. Jim asked to hold the baby, and ended up holding him for the entire time they were at the breakfast. Colleen remembered, "He kept coming up to me and saying, 'Let's sneak out the back door with the baby. We could just go now.'" Jim recalled, "I didn't want to let go of him, he was so beautiful. I had been dreaming about him for a long time. This was the boy I had dreamt of playing catch with when he was older. I hoped all day that the dream could come true."

In April, Jim and Colleen started taking the training seminar. Colleen remembered, "In the class we had four social workers, plus a social worker who was one of the instructors, plus the foster mother and her husband whom we had met at the fundraiser. There were four other couples attending the classes. The important thing to know, however, was that in the twelve weeks of the class the baby that the foster couple was caring for was always there, and Jim kept getting more and more attached. When we would drive home Jim would say, "Wouldn't it be nice if we'd get Aaron?"

At about this time, Nicole was feeling abandoned by Doctor D. During the three months on Clomid, she remembered, "He gave me the prescription and then basically just left me on my own. When the Clomid didn't work, he wanted to do a diagnostic laparoscopy. I felt lost; I didn't really know the purpose of the surgery or the results he hoped for. Up to that point I had not been aggressively researching on my own, so I didn't know what questions to ask. I was really putting myself in his hands, and he made no attempts to help me."

Nicole had the surgery in May, and it was a turning point for her and Jason. Jason recalled, "I felt that he would find an answer by doing the surgery. Months and months had passed without anything happening, and it was really frustrating. I wanted a baby and at the same time was being bombarded by these feelings of desperation. What was bad was when I'd watch a TV commercial that showed a dad holding his newborn baby in the air, or look outside and see my neighbor pitching balls to his son. Fatherhood was something I could only dream about. It's hard to see that stuff, and you see it every day."

Jason and Nicole's mother, Nancy, accompanied Nicole to the hospital. She had the laproscopic procedure that day. After the nurse took Nicole to be prepped for surgery, she came back and told her husband and mother that the procedure would take about forty-five minutes. The nurse said that after the procedure, Jason and Nancy would be brought to Doctor D's office. She told them they should wait until the doctor came so he could explain how the surgery had gone. Jason said, "After forty-five minutes passed they put us in his office. Another forty-five minutes passed, and he still hadn't come. I went out and asked the nurse what the problem was. She told me that she thought he had left the building. Then she checked her records and told me that he was still in surgery because there had been a problem with a woman he was doing a laparoscopy on. I thought, *Oh my God.* The nurse went to make sure, and then told me that Nicole was in recovery. She told us to wait for twenty minutes and then we could see her. We hadn't eaten—we were starving and we couldn't leave. A half-hour later Nancy got up and stormed over to the nurse's desk and demanded to know what was going on. It was at that point that we found out that Nicole hadn't even gone into surgery yet. The woman that was in recovery was named Nicole, too.

"We were so upset and worried. It was another hour after that before they told us Nicole was done and we could see her. We were so angry, and had lost faith in the people who were supposed to be taking care of Nicole. Nancy and I finally did see the doctor. We saw him for five minutes, tops."

The doctor explained to Jason and Nancy that Nicole had a few small ovarian cysts and some mild endometriosis. He surmised that Jason and Nicole were one of the few couples who had unexplained infertility problems—nothing appeared to be causing a problem with their fertility. Nicole said, "The doctor really pushed this 'wait and see' attitude. He said I should stop worrying about getting pregnant. He told me that he had this patient who was just like me: unexplained infertility. He told me that after five years she woke up pregnant one day and then had a baby. He really didn't dwell on options. He mentioned in vitro fertilization (IVF) as a possibility, but felt I should just wait to see what would happen. I was so emotionally confused that I didn't know if I was ready for the new technologies, so I never asked him to explain it any further."

Colleen and Jim had their final adoption training session in July. The session was held at their home, and was a counseling experience. While this was going on, Jim and Colleen received a call telling them that Aaron was going to be placed with them. Colleen remembered, "We really were unhappy with our new case worker. Ever since we met Aaron and his foster parents, we really wanted to adopt him. Had the foster parents not known us and had we not communicated as well as we did, I don't think the placement would have occurred. I think the foster mother is the only reason that we have Aaron today. The social worker on our case kept telling us that she had had other parents picked out for Aaron, and that we should be grateful we got him."

Aaron was placed as a fost/adopt, legal risk child. What this meant was that Aaron was to be a foster child with Colleen and Jim until the adoption ruling was finalized. The agency had done all of the parental rights termination proceedings prior to the placement of Aaron in the couple's home, but the appeal process for the birth parents had not yet ended.

On the last hour of the last day, the birth mother appealed the termination. Colleen remembered, "It was such a shock. We had known that the state had three months to file their legal briefs, and we had been given that time frame to expect a ruling. But the foster parents had planned going on vacation on the first of August, and their goal had been for the placement to be done by then. We had literally done the whole thing by ourselves. The worker was at their house with us just once for visitation. The day that we went and got him, the child protection worker who had been assigned to the case earlier and who no longer had any responsibility came and did the placement for us, because our worker didn't have the time. She brought a cake and presents, and I think had she not done those symbolic things, well, I know what would have happened. We would have gone and picked him up and the foster parents would have been grieving. Even as it was, I can still remember walking out the door and hearing the foster mother sobbing. It was uncomfortable enough to leave that day. I don't know if we would have ever left had that worker not been there to help us. We'd probably still be standing in that living room trying to leave."

Colleen stayed home with her son for a month, and then began taking him to his previous foster parents for daycare. Colleen said, "Aaron was a special needs child, and has suffered severe brain trauma from abuse. Aaron would wake every half hour with night terrors, so his foster parents had spent a lot of time with him and helped him through his therapies. They are still involved in the therapy, and in everything we have done with him. I think it made for a really healthy placement, because he never had to break those bonds. They became another grandma and grandpa to Aaron." After all Colleen and Jim had been through, however, there was still a chance that his birth mother's appeal could mean losing him.

After the laparoscopy, Nicole decided not to return to Doctor D. His condescending attitude and unwillingness to aggressively look for answers to their infertility was more than enough to make Nicole leave his care. A few months later, the couple was told that Colleen and Jim had Aaron placed in their home. Jason remembered, "It was such a difficult time for us. When we heard about the placement, we were very jealous. We were happy for them, but sad for us. There were times when they would come to town and I wouldn't want to see them with their son because it was too painful. I've never told anyone except Nicole."

It was at this point that Nicole started researching their options. She said, "I'd looked at IVF, but it scared me because of the cost and the complexity of the procedure. As I researched it I found out there were a lot more steps than I thought, and that the success rate was rather low. I thought about adopting from a state agency, but since my mom had been an adoption specialist and my sister had just had a child placed, I knew what we would be up against. In my opinion, our chances were slim to none of getting a normal, healthy baby.

"We looked into international and private adoption. I contacted two lawyers about it. But then we arrived at that awful barrier: cost. I kept asking, 'How do we pay for that?' The costs I was quoted ranged from seventy-five hundred to thirty thousand dollars. Were we supposed to go to the bank and offer our adopted child as collateral? It seemed like there weren't any options.

"As I started researching independent adoptions, I knew I would have to figure out how to pay for it, so I wondered if I was up to placing ads and trying to sell ourselves to a birth mom. I couldn't imagine myself trying to explain why I wanted her child. Trying to prove ourselves was so overwhelming. It's frustrating because you think, *Why should I have to prove myself to be a mother? No one else does.* When you are infertile it feels like your life is always in someone else's hands."

Nicole and Jason's marriage had become very rocky from all of the stress they had endured. The couple knew that they really needed to find some outlet for their emotions. Nicole said, "I felt Jason didn't know enough or care enough about how upset I was or about how I feared our infertility. I always did the reading and the research—I did it all. Then he expected me to tell him what I found. I resented that expectation. I felt I was carrying more of the burden around."

Jason also admitted to feeling resentment. He said, "Nicole would research adoption options and she wouldn't tell me about them. I was interested, but I just didn't want to research. My first choice was for a biological baby, so maybe that added to my not wanting to research adoption by myself.

"Sometimes I would also resent her depression. She would be down and I would want to do something, and she would refuse. I needed a way to blow off infertility. I tried to get her to talk to me about her feelings, but she wouldn't. She doesn't share her feelings readily."

Speaking up about infertility and the feelings that it evokes can be very difficult, especially for the person who has been diagnosed with the fertility problem. Nicole said, "Infertility is the most sensitive subject I have ever dealt with. When you open yourself up to somebody and you don't get a response, it is wounding. Sometimes I felt that people—including Jason at times—thought I should get on with it, get over it, and shut up about it.

"I did eventually find people to talk with. I confided in a couple of women at work. That was really good for me, because before that, work was a hellish place. It helped that they weren't family. One thing I found very comforting was that I had a friend who told me she couldn't imagine being in my shoes. She said, 'I never even thought about infertility when I got married. Now that I am learning about your experience I have no idea of what to say to you or even what I should feel for you.' To me that was the most open and honest thing anyone ever told me." Nicole found great comfort in her friend's honest reaction. By being so frank, her friend validated Nicole's experience with infertility. Her sentiment was sincere, and she never offered glib advice.

As Colleen and Jim waited for the result of the appeal and the news that the adoption was finalized, they heard a rumor that Aaron's birth mother was pregnant and that his birth father had robbed a business and been taken into custody. Colleen remembered, "As all of this was going on we were in a constant dialogue with the agency, trying to find out what was going to happen to the baby. They basically left us in the dark for a long time and never told us anything. They finally told us their goal was to take the baby from the birth mother. They asked if we would be interested in taking the baby into foster care, because the state's philosophy is to keep siblings together.

"We really agonized over that; it was a tough decision to make. They more or less said that if we didn't take the baby as a foster child, we'd lose our chance of ever having it placed with us. At the same time, however, they made sure we understood that there were no guarantees.

"The birth mother had a boy, Linc, in May of 1992. We spent that whole weekend sitting at home, not talking on the phone, not doing anything because we were waiting for the call to pick up the baby. It was all arranged with the sheriff that they were going to take the baby from the nursery and bring him to us. Tired of waiting, Jim called the worker that was assigned to the case and she said, 'I don't know what's happening.' She called the hospital and found out that the doctor had decided he wasn't going to let the baby go until Monday."

The waiting put a terrible strain on the couple. Monday morning Jim and Colleen met the social worker at the agency and picked up baby Linc. Colleen remembered, "I had such mixed feelings, because half the people we talked to were telling us this was a sure thing and that the birth mother would never get the baby back, and the other half were advising us not to get our hopes up. While we had been waiting, someone had asked us what his name was, and I said, 'I don't know.' And now as I look back on it I realize that I had known his name. I think it was my way of saying that I wanted this child; we had told no one we were going to get the baby because we were afraid of the birth parents finding us, and I suppose I was being extra careful by not giving his name. The last thing I said when we walked out the door of the agency was, 'Call the county sheriff's office and tell them that if they get a strange call in the middle of the night, they know where to go.'"

The couple had taken Aaron to daycare and had used Nancy's car to pick up Linc. After they had the child in their care, they went to Nancy's home. Jim and Colleen had been there for about twenty minutes when the phone rang. The call was from the adoption supervisor at the agency, asking the couple to come in and see her. Colleen recalled, "She had been in court when we picked up Linc. We went to her office and she said, 'I just wanted to remind you that this is a foster care situation and not to get your hopes up.'" The supervisor was emotionless as she told the couple about the weekly visitations the birth mother would be making. The visitations were scheduled for three times a week, and each would last two hours.

After Linc had been with them for a while, Colleen and Jim realized the true consequences of their decision. Colleen remembered, "Aaron's foster mother, knowing what these birth parents were like, helped us prepare for the visits. I was working full-time with a new baby, and Jim was not one to get up at night. I was really getting tired, and those visits were absolutely excruciating. It was unbelievable that we had to send that child on those visits to a woman who had severely abused her first child."

Linc had been in their home for three months before they got the call that the judge had ordered that Linc be returned to his birth mother. Colleen said, "We had planned a camping trip for the weekend, so I was at home that day with Aaron and Linc packing to go camping. At two in the afternoon the supervisor called and told me that the judge ordered that Linc be returned that day. I was hysterical as I called my mom and Jim. I don't even know in what order I called people. We had until six in the evening to be with him, so the whole family was over here. We gave him his last bath, and he rolled over for the first time. And then they came and got him, and we haven't seen him since. It was so hard because it was like a death, only you know the person is still alive and out there, but you are not allowed to ever see them again. During the time that this was going on, Aaron's adoption wasn't finalized either. We were panicking. Our whole life had turned upside down."

That Fall, Nicole talked with a friend of hers named Amanda. Amanda was also infertile and suggested that Nicole see her physician, Doctor E. Nicole and Jason talked about it and decided to call for an appointment. The nurse told Nicole that Doctor E was not taking new patients, but that Doctor F, an associate of his, was. Nicole agreed to see him, and the nurse told her that the doctor wanted both the husband and the wife present for the initial visit. Jason recalled, "No other doctor had ever wanted to see me before. The first and last time I ever met Doctor D was the day of Nicole's surgery, and that conversation lasted about five minutes. When we got there I immediately felt comfortable with him." Nicole remembered, "He sat down with both of us and talked for a long time. He asked about my past history, discussed the different types of infertility and ways to treat them, and then told me what his game plan would be for the first few months. He did a pelvic exam and advised Jason to be checked again. He told us we would start simple and then build up from there. He was very cautious, and checked everything."

Nicole started charting her temperature, went in for postcoital tests, and had a lot of blood work done. Early on, the doctor told the couple that a laparoscopy would probably not be necessary. But as he checked Doctor D's medical notes, he became worried. He told the couple he could not understand the notes, but that he would see if a video of the surgery was taken. When he called to see if a video was available, however, he was told one had not been done. Nicole recalled, "Doctor F couldn't believe there was not a videotape. He told me he wanted to do an x-ray of my tubes to make sure they were open, and that he needed to do a laparoscopy to feel confident that there was nothing else to do, because the tests weren't finding anything wrong. He was so patient, sincere, and really seemed to care about us. He always talked about options, costs, and even emotional feelings that were associated with each of the options. He brought up adoption, which was a subject no other doctor had even broached. I told him I would do the x-ray, but was not sure of the laparoscopy. He never pushed us into making a rash decision."

After the visit, Nicole went home deflated by the news. To even think about another laparoscopy was overwhelming to her. That evening her mother called to inquire about her health. Nicole said, "I was so crushed and my mom called and asked what the doctor had said. I just started bawling uncontrollably. All she could say was, 'I'm sorry.' I wanted her to say or do more. I wanted her to say, 'I'll give you ten thousand dollars to do an independent adoption. I will do the work for you, because it is so tough. I really needed someone to take care of me, but I know she didn't volunteer because she wanted us to be adults and go through the decision-making process. We would get to a barrier and I would ask her how we could go about getting a loan for an adoption, hoping she would offer to help. All she would say is, 'I don't know.' It seemed she was putting me up against more obstacles, and I wondered why."

Nicole was not the only sister to notice her mother's seeming disinterest in helping with an adoption. Colleen said, "I know that when Nicole was considering adoption, every time she asked my mother a question, my mother would give her an incredibly vague answer. Both Nicole and I looked into private adoptions, and when we would go to mom with questions the answers were always very general and not readily given. I think she was holding back because she knew what could happen to prospective adoptive parents—the pain they had to endure when the child was placed and then later returned to the birth parents."

In November, Nicole scheduled an appointment to have her tubes checked for obstructions. Since Colleen was going to the city that day, Nicole suggested they could go together. Nicole remembered, "The test was so painful, and I left the clinic in tears. Colleen seemed so uncomfortable being with me. I was hoping she would say something to me; it was really awkward." The doctor had told Nicole that there seemed to be a blockage, but without a laparoscopy he could not be sure. He had explained that sometimes the x-ray gives the impression that the tubes are blocked when they actually are not.

The doctor also explained that there is a small canal that connects the uterus to the tubes, and that it will constrict at times to slow down the passage of sperm trying to get in the tube. He further explained that the dye which had been used in the test may not have been able to get beyond the uterus because of such a constriction. Nicole remembered, "When I left I didn't know if I should be happy or if I was back at square one again. I told the doctor that I would need time to consider whether I would proceed with the laparoscopy or not."

In December of that year, Colleen and Jim still had not heard a word about Aaron's adoption finalization. Colleen recalled, "I was so frustrated with the system that I called the deputy attorney general and explained the situation. He was absolutely ugly with me on the phone. I told him the state's briefs had been filed a year earlier. He argued with me about when the briefs were filed and about the length of time we had waited. Finally he conceded that I was right, but he was very snotty. He said, 'Well, I can't call up the state supreme court and tell them they have been holding up a child for over a year—they think they're God over there.' And that was the end of the conversation; he said good-bye and hung up. So I wrote a sugar-coated thank-you letter and sent a picture of Aaron along, just to let him know that Aaron is a real child and needed attention."

One reason Colleen and Jim were very anxious to get the finalization was that until it was done, they could not leave the state without obtaining permission. Until the adoption was finalized, the state retained guardianship of Aaron. Colleen said, "No one understands the desperation of wanting a child except those who are desperate. During this time, one of my employee's sisters found out she was pregnant and she didn't know what to do. The employee kept talking to me about the situation. Finally I told her that if her sister was interested in giving the child up, Jim and I would be interested in parenting. It was an incredible disappointment when she decided to give the baby to the state as a normal, healthy infant to be adopted by someone lucky enough to be on the waiting list.

"The insensitive things people do and say amazed me. I can remember everybody who ever said something insensitive to me, down to who said what, where, when, and even what they were wearing. The questions that have bothered me the most have been when people have asked us why we adopted and don't have our 'own' kids, and when they've asked how much Aaron cost us. Those hurt, and you don't get over them."

In January, Nicole and Jason decided to have one more infertility procedure done. They called Doctor F and scheduled the laparoscopy. The couple kept their plans a secret up until the night before the surgery. Jason took Nicole to the hospital, and after Nicole was in recovery, Doctor F asked Jason to come to his office and watch the video of the surgery with him. Jason remembered, "I was kind of taken aback, and the doctor asked me if I was comfortable watching the tape. I told him that we would find out. The intern, nurse, the doctor, and I watched the video, and he was explaining things the entire time. He pointed out the ovary and the tubes, keeping an eye on me to make sure I wasn't turning white. He told me everything looked normal. He answered all of my questions and was really great to talk to."

When Nicole woke up from the anesthetic, Jason explained what the doctor had told him. Jason recalled, "She said there had to be something wrong. Nicole asked if her tubes were blocked, and I told her the doctor didn't find any blockage. She wouldn't believe me, so we called the nurse. The nurse had the doctor come to the phone, and he explained there wasn't anything wrong. He told her that the dye went through the tubes freely. I could tell Nicole was relieved, but I think she was also bothered by him not finding a cause for our infertility."

That evening, Jason and Nicole brought the video over to Nancy's house and asked Nancy, Jim, and Colleen to view the surgery with them. Colleen remembered, "We had to draw the line when they wanted us to watch the videotape of the surgery. Even when visiting with people who have dealt with infertility, I find myself feeling uncomfortable with it. One of the couples we know is very free in talking about the procedures and surgeries they have had, and I find myself very uncomfortable hearing that. It was like they were opening their medical history up to me. I didn't want to hear about it. I don't know if it was that I didn't want to acknowledge that I, too, might be in the same situation, or what."

In February, both couples and Nancy went to DisneyWorld for a much-needed vacation. In March, Nicole went back to her doctor for a checkup, and her period was five days late. The doctor said, "Wouldn't it be neat if you were pregnant?" But the pregnancy test she took the following week came back negative. Nicole said, "I had no symptoms. I remember that after the checkup I had heartburn once, but attributed it to eating one too many pieces of pizza.

"Jason was out of town when I missed the next cycle in April. I started wondering when I went to the grocery store whether I should go down 'that' aisle; the aisle where the pregnancy kits are. I thought, *I'm not going to set myself up for that heartbreak.* Finally, on a Thursday evening, I decided to pick one up. I thought the test would be negative and would give me a reason to go and bitch at my doctor. I brought home the test, took it, and when I checked the result, it was positive! I remember screaming, I was so excited. But then that little voice kicked in and said, *Well, you probably did it wrong.* So I read the instructions again and thought I'd better buy another one to be sure. It was positive too, and I was ecstatic. I couldn't sleep that night. I was all alone and I didn't call anybody. I wanted to savor it and keep it all to myself. I went to bed that night with the biggest smile on my face, thinking, *My God, it's finally going to happen.*"

The next day was Good Friday, and Nicole tried to get a doctor's appointment for that afternoon to have her pregnancy confirmed. The clinic told her it was impossible and that she would have to wait until the following week. In the meantime, Jason arrived home after driving twenty-four hours straight from Mississippi. Jason remembered, "I called her at work and told her, 'I'm home, I'm exhausted, and I'm going to sleep.' A little later she was at my side, telling me to get up because she had this early Easter present for me. I opened it and I found a book of baby names, along with the positive pregnancy test. As I saw it I said, 'Oh my God, is it true?' We were both jumping with excitement."

The couple decided to keep their pregnancy a secret from Nicole's family until Easter Sunday. Jason said, "I called everyone on my side right away. I called my mom, brother, and even my grandparents. I was flying high and I had to share the news. We told them we had no idea why we had gotten pregnant at last, we were just glad we had."

On Saturday, Jason and Jim went Easter shopping for their wives. Jim recalled, "We went to buy porcelain figurines, but Jason wouldn't let me see which figure he got. I thought he must not trust me to keep the secret from Colleen until Easter, which was weird because Easter was the next day. We never dreamed Nicole was pregnant—after all, she had just had surgery."

Easter Sunday arrived, and Nicole handed out Easter baskets. Colleen remembered, "She gave us all Easter baskets, and each had a baby item in it. I got a baby bottle, Mom a pacifier, and Jim had a bib in his basket. That's when they made the announcement. My first thoughts were, *Why can't it be me?* but I was crying because I was happy for her."

In May, Aaron's birth mother was prosecuted on criminal child abuse charges. Colleen said, "I don't think we are over the experience with Linc. After we heard about the birth mom, we knew something was going to happen. I think we lived a false dream that he was coming back, and we didn't let ourselves get over it until we knew that it wasn't going to happen. The state approached us about whether we would take him back as a foster child again, and we decided we couldn't do that to ourselves or Aaron. For the first few weeks after Linc left, when Aaron saw a baby, he would ask if it was baby Linc. Now all we have is a picture to show Aaron. For us, all that is left of Linc are our pictures."

The following month, almost two years after Aaron was placed, Colleen and Jim finalized his adoption. Colleen said, "At the finalization we talked to the worker, and she asked us if we were going to put in our order for another child. I told her we needed a period of time where we weren't dealing with the agency. And since Nicole announced her pregnancy, mom has been telling me, 'You need to go to the doctor too.' When I respond by saying that we need time to live a normal life for awhile, she tells me that I am in denial and that I'll never get pregnant because I will never go to the doctor.

"Adoption fills the parenting need for us. Rocking Aaron in the middle of the night and singing to him fills an intense need of mine. He will always be our baby, but there is still a desire to have a baby. We think we are almost ready to see the doctor now. Jim's clock is ticking—he will be forty this year." Jim agreed and said, "My mom was forty-two when I was born. I never wanted to be too old to play catch in the yard with my kids. If that is to happen, we need to have another child sometime soon."

As Colleen and Jim struggle to make decisions, they wonder what is in their future. Colleen said, "Aaron has taken the desperation and urgency that I felt to have another baby away. I do have a newfound desire to conceive now that Nicole is pregnant. I also know that Jim, Aaron, and I need to rest before we do something else. We don't want to think about adoption or trying to conceive a child at least for a little while. I think that time will come very soon, though."

Colleen and Nicole have faced their infertility in different ways: Colleen chose adoption, while Nicole went through infertility treatments. Happily, Colleen has an adopted child and, at the time this is being written, Nicole is expecting her baby.

During their interviews, the sisters offered advice on surviving adoption and surviving infertility treatments. Interestingly enough, the advice was the same: ask questions, don't accept answers at face value, and keep fighting the system.

3

Shared Infertility

BARS

I don't want the bars anymore—
please take them away.
They've hurt me from heart to core;
I fear they are here to stay.

I'm a prisoner, not by choice,
unless my memory serves me wrong.
I can hear my children's voices
I can sing to them my song.

Rock a bye baby in the treetop
you never came down to form in my womb.
Rock a bye baby, why did you stop?
you died as a whisper, my sweet dreams your tomb.

I don't want the bars anymore—
was my faith just too weak?
I fasted, wept, and prayed to God daily before—
the bars are a void, black and bleak.

I don't want the bars anymore—
I never really did.
I can hardly open that door and
look at that crib.

Rock a bye baby in the treetop
you never came down to form in my womb.
Rock a bye baby why did you stop
you died as a whisper, my sweet dreams your tomb.

I don't want the bars anymore—
so get rid of that crib.
I know it's a chore,
so don't wait 'till high bid.

I don't want the bars anymore—
the disassembled package sell.
See if there is a buyer from the paper or store.
We'll keep it a secret, and I'll never tell.

Those bars, they block me—
they are there downstairs.
Those crib bars stand at attention
between the lambies and bears.

Rock a bye baby in the treetop
you never came down to form in my womb.
Rock a bye baby, why did you stop?
you died as a whisper, my sweet dreams your tomb.

I don't want the bars anymore—
please take them away.
They've hurt me from heart to core;
I fear they are here to stay.

Those bars were a dream
in a pitiful game.
I never knew such devotion
could turn, twist, and maim,
that tears would scatter
over crib quilt clothes
and the smell of baby lotion.

Rock a bye baby in the treetop
you never came down to form in my womb.
Rock a bye baby, why did you stop?
You died as a whisper, my sweet dreams your tomb.

I don't want the bars anymore—
please take them away.
They've hurt me from heart to core
I fear they are here to stay.

This poem was written by Sara, who at the time was being haunted by a baby crib she had bought. Every time Sara went into the basement she saw the little crib. At first it symbolized hope and innocence. As time passed, however, and she struggled with infertility and mourned the babies she had lost, the crib came to represent a malignancy. The beautiful little crib taunted her unmercifully, and the poem "Bars" evolved from that experience. Sara said, "We bought the crib after we had been struggling with infertility for quite awhile. We bought it hoping I'd get pregnant, or that we could use it for an adopted baby.

"It was really difficult to go into the room with the crib in it after awhile. I really started hating having it in the house. We sold it at a rummage sale to another infertile couple who had finally become pregnant. I remember showing the woman how the crib worked. As I was showing it to her I realized I never got to use it, and there I was showing her how it worked. It was very hard. They loaded the crib into this big old station wagon, and as they drove off I wanted to shout at them to bring it back."

Watching the couple drive away with the crib symbolically reinforced Kyle and Sara's infertility. They, as an infertile couple, were watching once again as other people began their lives as new parents. It was a cruel reminder of their plight.

Sara and Kyle had never dreamed infertility would be a part of their lives. They both came from large families and carried with them a strong love of children. Both came from very religious backgrounds. Sara's parents were missionaries in Japan, and Kyle's father was a Baptist Minister; their love of God and family was fostered very early on in their lives. As they entered into marriage they took their fertility for granted. They wanted children, but did not feel an overwhelming need to have a baby right away. Neither Sara's nor Kyle's parents had suffered from infertility, and it was a topic that was not discussed in their homes.

Sara and Kyle were married in December, and after their honeymoon they threw themselves into their work. Both felt that by working hard they could begin to establish a comfortable income level and feel a sense of accomplishment from doing their jobs well. Kyle worked days and Sara worked nights as they focused on building a nest egg. By the end of the following Spring, Sara was working close to seventy hours a week between several jobs.

At this point, Sara began to feel run down, and she realized her period was late by about two weeks. She did not know if she should attribute the feeling to exhaustion, or to the possibility of a pregnancy. Because she and her husband were not covered by medical insurance, Sara decided to postpone a doctor's visit.

A few days later she began experiencing severe back pain and started shaking, and as Kyle rushed her to the emergency room she started to go into shock. The doctor treated her for shock and diagnosed pelvic inflammatory disease (PID). PID is a medical condition that can cause adhesions on the reproductive organs, can cause scar tissue to form on the fallopian tubes, and can sometimes cause infertility. The doctor told her that he was unsure of what had caused the condition, and did not bother to share the information about the possible consequences of PID. He gave Sara a prescription for antibiotics and told her that if she would have had insurance, he would have hospitalized her for a few days. As it was, he told her to take the medication and rest at home.

Sara took the medication, but had a difficult time with the whole idea of staying inactive and resting. But since rest had been prescribed, she did just that. Sara remembered, "During this time a nephew was born. Being married only six months, we really weren't planning on a pregnancy, but after the PID I started thinking about having kids. We had not been using contraceptives, and I started wondering about our chances."

As the summer passed, Sara began having pain in her pelvic area. Concerned that she was having another bout with PID, she went to a gynecologist, Doctor B, to have an exam. Sara told him about the PID and described the pain she was feeling.

Upon doing a pelvic exam the doctor diagnosed an ovarian cyst, and told her he felt a thickening in her tubes. He advised Sara to have a cystectomy via a laparoscopy. He told her that a laparoscopy was a simple, same-day surgical procedure that would enable him to remove the cyst and to check for scarring or adhesions that may have been left from the PID. Then he suggested she watch a video at the clinic that explained the laproscopic procedure.

Sara remembered, "In the video they showed a woman who was cheerfully answering phones, and the voiceover announced that laparoscopy was a simple surgery—it would be fine to go back to work a few days afterward. I had the surgery, but as I recovered from the anesthesia I had very severe nausea. Still, because the doctor and the video suggested that work was plausible soon after the surgery, I went back to work waitressing after two days. You know, you never think about plates and food weighing that much, but I was hefting these huge platters of food and carrying crates of ketchup and things. I was totally exhausted. There were times that I felt I was going to pass out."

Six months passed, and Sara continued to have pelvic pains and irregular menstrual cycles. During that time, the couple had moved to a different town, so Sara made an appointment with a general practitioner, Doctor C, to see if he could find a way to relieve her pain. Doctor C listened to Sara's past medical history, and as he examined her he asked how much time had elapsed since the last laparoscopy. Sara told him it had been about six months since the procedure and then explained her experience of going back to work two days after the surgery.

Sara said, "He told me that my scar should not still be red, that he thought I overdid it, and that I probably had a lot of scar tissue as a result. As he did the pelvic exam he said he thought I might have a tubal pregnancy because of the lump he felt, and also because my period had been really late. He scheduled an ultrasound for the next morning and told me there was a possibility of a partial hysterectomy if I indeed did have a tubal pregnancy. I remember he told me this information very matter-of-factly. There was no compassion or empathy for my situation.

"The night before the ultrasound I got very little sleep. At twenty, the idea of a hysterectomy was very frightening. I was incredibly panicky. The next morning I went in for the ultrasound not knowing if he was going to find a tubal pregnancy or not. At that time I was pretty ignorant of how our bodies work, and up until this experience I had thought medicine was an exact science. This was the turning point for me that led to my questioning the medical treatment that was recommended to me.

"The doctor found that I had an ovarian cyst, but said it wasn't very large yet. He said there was not a tubal pregnancy; therefore a hysterectomy was not indicated. He recommended I see a gynecologist to see about getting the cyst removed.

"As I look back on my medical experiences, I have found that the best doctors are ones who listen to you. Prior to this experience, I had felt that nothing I had to say was valid. After all, what did I know about my body? All I knew was that it hurt."

Because of the tension and fear that had surrounded Sara's last medical experience, she put off seeing a gynecologist for a few months. Finally, Kyle suggested that she make the appointment to have the cyst removed. Sara went to Doctor D, a gynecologist in their new community, and once again explained her history and detailed the pain she had experienced.

As part of his medical workup the doctor asked Sara if she and Kyle were actively pursuing a pregnancy. Sara remembered, "The question would always be, 'Are you trying to have children or not?' Now, when I grew up, my parents never really *tried* to have children. I don't think they even used contraceptives, although the topic was never talked about. They had five children, and I know that my mother miscarried at least once. To me, the doctor's question was very personal. Whether we were trying to conceive or not was our business. I was appalled that he asked us that.

"The doctor removed the cyst and then gave us a little booklet on tips for conception. That was when the wheel started to turn around—this was the time when I truly started wondering if there was going to be a problem. As we talked about pregnancy I asked questions, but did not stress any urgency. The doctor's attitude at that point was very nonaggressive. He said, 'When you start trying to get pregnant, try for six months, and if you are not pregnant, come back to see me.'"

It was after this visit that Sara and Kyle decided it was time to start their family. Within a year after their decision, Sara believes she may have been pregnant and miscarried up to seven times. She remembered, "At that time I didn't know that I should chart my temperature, but my cycles were like clockwork. My cycles invariably had been twenty-eight days in length. With the first pregnancy I was about a month late, which would have made the fetus about six weeks old. I remember the day I miscarried very vividly.

"We were in our apartment and had gone to church that day. I definitely had symptoms; some nausea, some bloating. I didn't do a pregnancy test because I felt that if I made it past a month, then I would take the test. But at church and that morning, everything in the service affirmed the fact that I was pregnant. It was like every verse seemed to speak to me, and it was such a rewarding feeling.

"As I came out of the church I started feeling very severe cramping, and had a feeling like something had detached from my uterus, which I had never felt before. I told Kyle to take me home immediately.

"I lay down, and the blood began to pour out of my body. I knew this was definitely a pregnancy because I had never flowed like this before, even when I had been late. The amount and intensity of the flow frightened me. I lay in the fetal position and held my arms taut against my chest. I remember lying there wondering if I should go to the doctor, but I was still pretty ignorant about what to do. I felt if I did go in, I wouldn't know what questions I should ask. I had always known the basics of the human body and reproduction, but that was it.

"I called my parents and told them I was miscarrying, and they wept with me over the phone. I did not feel comfortable telling very many people, because Kyle's brother and wife were pregnant, as well as many of our friends. (It seems when you miscarry, everybody's pregnant.) We did tell Kyle's mom and dad. Telling his mom, Maria, was like putting it on a radio broadcast, because she told everybody. After Maria heard about the miscarriage, she called Kyle's sister Ellen. Ellen then called me and told me that I should really allow myself to grieve, that it was okay to grieve. At that point I really let myself cry—up until then I was tense and pretty numb. Somehow in my warped mind I thought that if I tensed up I would be able to hold onto this baby."

Sara believes that she will forever feel the grief of her miscarriage: "Every time I drive by the apartment where I miscarried, I feel like a very important piece of me got left there."

A few months passed, and Sara tried to bury the emotional turmoil she had faced by throwing herself into her work. But then, she said, "I was about twelve days late with my cycle, and I had begun to experience the nausea and had breast tenderness. I was coming back from some kind of committee that I was on, and as I was sitting in the car I felt something drop and let loose from me. I got up, and the seat of the car was covered with blood. I didn't know what to do."

As Sara stood staring at the bloody seat, her hand went to her mouth, and she gasped at the thought that she was losing another baby. As a way of protecting her emotional stability, however, Sara began telling herself that these were just periods. She remembered, "It got to the point that when I was late with my cycle and had pregnancy symptoms, I would deny the possibility I was pregnant. Then when I would start to bleed it would come in huge clots and I would lose massive amounts of blood. To protect my sanity, I found myself thinking that all the bleeding was now normal for me. I would flow through two super maxipads and a super tampon within a short amount of time, and I began to think this was normal. I know now that every time this happened—probably about seven times within the year—that I was pregnant, and that I did miscarry. At the time I would have never admitted that I was having that many miscarriages to anyone—even myself. The horror of that realization would have been too difficult to bear."

Then Sara's sister, Beth, gave birth to a baby. Beth and her husband Todd had fought infertility for seven years before a pregnancy had been achieved. Sara remembered, "At the time of the birth I was having so many problems dealing with the pain and grief of infertility. The most healing thing I experienced was when my sister invited me to come right after the birth and help take care of the baby. It was so healing to be able to care for that baby. I loved the fact that I could hold this tiny newborn at any time of the day."

As the year ended, Sara began to notice that the last few cycles she had experienced were not late, and the heavy bleeding had dramatically decreased. During this time Sara visited a friend named Kim. During their conversation, Kim disclosed her own struggle with infertility. She told Sara that she was seeing Doctor E, a reproductive endocrinologist in another town. Kim and her husband Bob were very pleased with the doctor, because he seemed to be very interested in working with them to find answers to their infertility. Sara then discussed this news with Kyle, and they decided to make an appointment. The fact that he was a reproductive endocrinologist appealed to the couple, because he would be able to determine if their infertility was partly caused by hormonal problems.

Months later, Sara and Kyle's appointment date arrived. They felt nervous, yet were relieved that the time to find answers had finally come. Sara and Kyle were very pleased that the doctor specifically asked to see the couple together on the initial visit. He explained what he planned to do for the infertility workup, and he asked about Sara's past gynecological history.

As she told him of her experiences with the late cycles and the heavy bleeding, Sara felt a huge burden being lifted off her shoulders. The doctor listened to her story and told her that she very well could have been pregnant each one of those times and then gone on to miscarry the babies. He said it sounded like she had been able to conceive at that point in time, but that her womb might be unable to accept implantation.

The endocrinologist then did a pelvic exam on Sara. After he had finished, he told Sara to get dressed and then to come into his office, where he would discuss his findings with her and her husband. Sara remembered, "He gave us rather tragic news. He found extreme swelling of the tubes on one side. In doing the pelvic he felt that there was a possibility the fimbria on my fallopian tubes weren't extending, and that there was a possibility I was not ovulating. He told me to chart my basal body temperature so we could determine if I was ovulating. He wanted me to chart my temperature for four months, and each month I would come in for a postcoital test. After the four months, the doctor felt it might be necessary to perform a laparotomy before further diagnosis." Sara was told that a laparotomy would require an incision in the abdomen and a recovery period both at the hospital and at home.

As the doctor gave them his findings he very carefully explained in detail what each of his findings meant. He explained that each month a woman's body should produce an egg from one of the ovaries. At the point of ovulation, the egg is released from one of the ovaries into the abdominal cavity. It is at this point that the fallopian tubes try to retrieve the egg. They can do this because at the end of the tube is a wide, flower-like opening, called the fimbria. The fimbria, after the egg is extruded from the ovary, reaches out for the egg and draws the egg into the tube. The egg travels through the tube and is either fertilized or disintegrates. The doctor felt that instead of her fimbria being open, they had closed in on themselves.

Sara remembered thinking, *How can an egg get in there?* Then came the realization that it would be very difficult, if not impossible, for the egg to make it into one of her tubes.

The doctor then went on to explain that the next step would be to determine if she indeed was ovulating. He could determine this by reading Sara's basal body temperature charts. He explained that she would need to take her temperature at the same time each morning before getting out of bed. He then showed the couple an example of a normal chart and demonstrated how to record her daily temperature.

Doctor E also advised Kyle to get a sperm analysis done so Kyle's fertility could be determined. He told Kyle that he could have the test done in their home town clinic, so as to avoid traveling one hundred miles to have the test at the doctor's laboratory.

Oftentimes, infertility tests are less than natural procedures. Yet, men and women who have suffered through infertility for extended periods of time usually reach a point when the tests become a part of everyday life. Modesty over cooperating with them becomes a thing of the past. For Kyle, however, this was the first infertility test that he had to do.

Kyle remembered, "I felt that the method of getting a sperm sample was very demeaning. But I kept telling myself that Sara had already gone through so much that nothing compared to her experiences." The results that came back from the lab reported that the count was adequate. At the news, Kyle breathed a sigh of relief.

Meanwhile, Sara began taking her daily temperature, and the couple began going into the doctor's office to have postcoital tests taken. A postcoital test is one in which the doctor checks the woman's cervical mucus as well as the sperm's ability to penetrate that mucus. (Prior to ovulation, a woman's cervix opens and secretes thick cervical mucus to help facilitate the sperm's journey to the uterus.) This test is performed as close to ovulation as possible. A couple is instructed to have intercourse, and two hours later the doctor takes a sample of the mucus and examines it under the microscope to see if there are sperm moving freely within the mucus.

Sara said of that experience, "At the time he started doing the post-coital tests, it was a very difficult period for us. Having our sex life scheduled and being told when we had to have sex and when we could not was humiliating. But we got to a point where we started to joke about the lack of control. We would come in for the test and sit in the waiting room full of people as the nurse would come over and ask us what time we had intercourse. We started laughing about it and being very open with each other. I think this has to happen before you can be open with other people about infertility."

As Sara and Kyle pursued their dream for a baby, they experienced the intense grief that is a natural part of infertility. At the time, however, neither knew that their feelings were normal. Sara remembered, "Each month I would start grieving even before my cycle would start. It was difficult for me to remember what it felt like to be happy. I would play all these mind games with myself. One of the games I played was buying a jumbo package of tampons. By doing so, I reasoned, I would ensure I would not need them. I played games with God as well. I had been told that caffeine consumption really reduces the chances of a pregnancy occurring, and there would be days I would consume caffeine to spite Him. I would rant to God about the injustice of my infertility, somehow thinking a private colloquy would change His will."

Sara's faith in God was truly tested by her war with infertility. When individuals begin to question the very core beliefs of their lives, they begin to feel overwhelming amounts of guilt for doing so, and Sara was no exception. When she began to question why she had to live with infertility, she felt her self-esteem was affected. She said, "It affected my self-esteem because I have always been a go-getter in whatever I have done. To not be able to have a baby really hurt. The aching to hold a child and the yearning to produce a miracle was not possible because of my physical condition. I view my infertility as a handicap, one that is not perceived visually. People don't understand the pain that goes on inside, and by that I am handicapped."

After four cycles of taking her basal body temperature and having post-coital tests without any clear indication of the source of Sara and Kyle's infertility, the laparotomy procedure was scheduled. The laparotomy differed from a laparoscopy in that it was, by any standard, a major surgery.

Instead of the tiny incision made to accommodate the thin tube used in a laproscopic procedure, a larger incision was made in Sara's abdomen to allow the doctor to make a further diagnosis and to remove any cysts or adhesions. After surgery, while Sara was in recovery, she asked to see her husband, Kyle. The medical staff searched for him, but were unable to locate him right away. Kyle recalled, "They were looking for me in the waiting room, but I wasn't there. I was so scared and nervous; I was in the men's bathroom, throwing up."

After Sara began to come out of the anesthesia, the doctor discussed the results of the laparotomy with the couple. He told them that he had used microsurgery to open the tubes, removed a large ovarian cyst from the right ovary, and removed several small clusters of cysts from her left ovary. He told Sara that when she did indeed ovulate, it was happening late in the cycle. He said she would be given FSH (follicle stimulating hormone) shots to help stimulate the follicle into developing; the fertility drug Clomid to increase the pituitary's production of FSH; and progesterone suppositories to ensure cervix closing after ovulation, and to aid in implantation of the embryo.

Sara said, "I get so nervous before surgeries because I'm such an 'eebie jeebie' person around hospitals. I'm terrified of what they will find out, and I always ask the doctor to come in and talk to me right away. I may not remember much of it because I'm still coming out of the anesthesia, but Kyle always remembers. I do remember when Doctor E came in to talk to us after my laparotomy and told me I was pretty much a mess. I was still groggy from the anesthesia, and I just started bawling. But I wanted to know the news as soon as possible so I didn't have to invent a diagnosis. My own diagnosis would probably be worse."

Around the time of her laparotomy, Sara's sister-in-law, Myra, got pregnant. At this point, Sara and Kyle were in the process of grieving their infertility and trying to keep themselves on an even emotional keel. To find out that Myra was pregnant after all that they had come through was difficult but manageable for the couple. What was harder to deal with was that Myra had announced to their church's congregation that even though she and her husband had gotten married after Sara and Kyle, she had gotten pregnant before them. Sara recalled, "I just couldn't believe she did that. That was, for me, the most killing thing. How she could be so insensitive just eluded me.

"Later I told Myra how her comments had hurt. I told my sister-in-law to be honest with me, but she did not have to treat me like I was made of eggshells. I told her, 'If I want to cry, let me cry on your shoulder—but please, don't turn your shoulder away.' I had known that if there are things she can't control, she doesn't know how to handle it. That was her approach to our infertility. If there have been one person's comments which I have been consistently hurt by, they have been hers. She speaks before she realizes she is putting her foot in her mouth."

At first, Kyle never really processed the insensitivities that he heard concerning their infertility. He said, "I never really was that in touch with my feelings—or Sara's—until recently. I started to become more aware of insensitive statements when I saw how they affected Sara. I can always tell how she has been hurt just by watching her. She pulls in her breath and becomes very quiet. Myra has inadvertently hurt Sara very deeply."

Another incident that affected Sara and Kyle took place when they invited a couple from church over for dinner. Sara recalled, "We had a new couple from church over for supper one night. They have children, and we were talking about children in general. We said we enjoyed our nephews and nieces, but enjoyed coming home to a quiet house. That was our way of saying 'we aren't having kids.' You just don't want to blurt out that you are infertile. It was a stupid way to do it, but we weren't going to unload on them.

"They just ripped us up one side and down the other. They advised us not to put it off. That really hurt. People don't mean to hurt, they just don't know any better."

To never have to hear insensitive remarks about infertility is a dream that most infertile people wish for. Intellectually, most infertile people realize others do not mean to hurt, but on an emotional level, careless comments can be powerful enough to tear an infertile person's heart out.

In the month following the laparotomy, the doctor did another post-coital test to determine if the medication Sara was on was helping her cervical mucus, and also to determine if she was ovulating. Sara remembered, "After I was on the medicine for a short time, my body pretty much went bizarre. My breasts were hurting all the time, I was nauseous, and it was incredibly stressful. It seemed like I was ovulating, but there was not a lot of cervical mucus apparent. And the postcoital test showed that

Kyle's sperm was not getting anywhere. The doctor invited Kyle to look under the microscope and view the sperm. It hurt me so much, because Kyle came back and he cried in my arms.

"This was a real turning point for us. It was no longer just my infertility that we were fighting; we now shared in the infertility. We wondered what we should do. We were very confused and were unsure if we should even continue treatment." At this point, however, Doctor E suggested artificial insemination using Kyle's sperm. The doctor told the couple that artificial insemination with Kyle's sperm would bypass Sara's lack of cervical mucus and get the slow-moving sperm directly into the uterus, where it would have a better chance of reaching the fallopian tubes.

Insemination is timed to occur during ovulation, and sexual intercourse is discouraged prior to and following ovulation in order to make the chances for conception optimal. The unfortunate side effect is that having one's sex life determined by a schedule can be very detrimental to the couple's feelings towards sex and intimacy. Kyle recalled, "At times the treatments made sex more of a medical procedure than an intimate bonding. It was no longer making love. It was not pleasurable at times. There were times we had sex just because the doctor told us we should do it."

Sara believes that their struggle with infertility had adverse effects on her feelings towards sexuality. She said, "We got off to a rough start sexually because of my past history. My parents were missionaries and I was, for the most part, raised in Japan. I went into marriage basically hating men, because my experience was that men are not real nice in Japan—white women are like prized possessions. So I came into the marriage with that attitude.

"Also, our sex life was not normal for a long time because it was physically painful and very frustrating for me. Even when I was on hormones for infertility I was not producing enough cervical mucus. It took me three years of marriage before I ever found out about lubricants. No one bothered to educate me and I thought the pain and frustration of sex was not worth it. I felt that I was not getting anything out of the experience and I really suffered in silence, because who do you talk to about such an intimate part of your life?

"One evening I was at my sister's home—she lives far away, so I felt I could talk to her. I asked her how many times, on average, normal couples had sex in a week. She told me she thought between two or three times a week. She saw my jaw fall open and asked me how often I was having sex. I told her maybe once a month. At that point I began to think we probably needed to go in for sexual counseling.

"Our problem worsened during our infertility treatments because our sex life was scheduled. There were times that I was travelling for my job when we should have been trying. I can't remember how many times I went in for a postcoital test or an artificial insemination on my way to the airport. How romantic! Then I had a hang-up with having sex at non-scheduled times because I would think that we would need to save the sperm up, or that I couldn't have sex because I wasn't ovulating yet. Infertility added so much stress and pressure. Between infertility and the demands of my job, it would be very easy to ignore each other and feel fulfilled in every aspect except sexuality. This is an area we have to work on."

Kyle and Sara went through two cycles of artificial insemination. Sara said of the experience, "It was a relatively simple procedure and did not cause the amount of stress the surgeries did. The doctor would do the insemination and then leave Kyle and me in the room to be together. It was an incredibly rewarding experience; it was nice to have that time to enjoy each other. I had to lie down for approximately twenty minutes after the insemination, and it was a nice time for Kyle and me to hold each other and dream about the possibility of becoming parents. I don't think this is a standard procedure, but we were grateful that our doctor encouraged it."

When a pregnancy did not result, the doctor referred Kyle to a urologist and told him that until his infertility was addressed, it was not advisable to continue artificial insemination. Kyle remembered, "I could handle the infertility when it was Sara who was having problems. Then I found out I was having problems too, and I felt so guilty. I have always had low self-esteem, so infertility did not knock it down too much more, but I did view myself differently. I felt that it was my fault that Sara couldn't get pregnant. She wanted a child so badly, and at times I thought that if I was dead she could get remarried and maybe have the child she dreamed of."

It was at this point that the couple started considering the possibility of adoption. As they talked about it, Kyle realized that although he knew families who had adopted, he never saw himself in the role of an adoptive father. Kyle said, "It took awhile for me to understand that I could accept and love an adopted child. My desire for a biological child was very strong, and it was hard to accept the realization that I might not be able to help create one."

Sara had a more positive reaction to adoption. She said, "I grew up always wanting to adopt children. When I was six, I was sent to boarding school. It was something like the experience of being in an orphanage, in that I did not know what was going on. I have always had empathy for children who are separated from their parents."

Soon after their first adoption discussion, Sara received a magazine that her church sent to its members. In the magazine was a section on special needs adoption written by a woman in Illinois. There were pictures of special needs children who were up for adoption, and a number to call if readers were interested in further information. Sara became very excited as she read the section and looked at the beautiful little faces in the pictures. She remembered, "I called the number and explained our infertility and the emotional problems it had caused. I told the woman that we had looked into private adoption for a newborn, that there were five- to seven-year waiting lists, and that the fees were very expensive. She told me that if we were willing to adopt a child with special needs, I should start at our own home base. She told me I should go to our town's social service agency and talk to an adoption worker."

Sara called the adoption specialist as soon as she got off the phone with the first woman. The specialist told Sara that she and Kyle could drop by any time to chat. Kyle and Sara were very excited, and went down the same day. Sara remembered, "Our adoption specialist was just wonderful. She was excited for us and showed us a three-ring binder full of new families who had successfully adopted. We told her that we were thinking about the possibility of adopting a special needs child, and she explained that there was a misnomer about the term 'special needs.' She said that to a lot of people, 'special needs' means a child who is mentally retarded or malformed, and this is not necessarily the case."

The adoption specialist explained that the adoption process was not a waiting list, but a process of matching children to families. The family who wanted to adopt needed to do a home study report, in which they listed their hobbies and interests as well as the types of special needs they would be willing to work with. Sara remembered, "There was lots of personal information, and they asked how much of a handicap we could handle. Completing the study was so emotionally wrenching to us. We would answer one page and then we would go for a walk and cry before doing the next page. Social services had told us that we had to be honest with ourselves. They told us that we needed to come to adoption with our expectations on the table. If you have dreams of a child becoming an astronaut and the child turns out to be a janitor, you need to be ready to adjust your expectations."

The couple met with their caseworker and then attended an intensive training workshop for people who wanted to become adoptive parents. Both Kyle and Sara were very impressed with the training they received. Kyle said, "It was one of the very best experiences I have had. Through the training, you really begin to acknowledge the grief that comes with the acceptance of the possibility of not being a biological parent. It also made me more open, more communicative with Sara about my feelings."

Through the home study and the training, Kyle and Sara decided that they could handle a child aged zero to three years of age, and would work with a child who had been emotionally or physically abused and/or neglected. Sara said, "I told them I could not handle a child who lied, cheated, or stole. I feel that Kyle and I are very good at being consistent disciplinarians, and that would enable us to nurture a child and give boundaries to a child who had none. I also said I could not handle a child who had been sexually abused or who was not legally free to be adopted. I think our requests had a lot to do with our infertility experiences."

After starting the adoption process, the couple made the decision that Kyle would see a urologist. Sara recalled, "It was weird being on the other end of infertility, because we had been married about five years, and for the first time it wasn't my problem. It was so odd not being the one to undergo surgery and not being the one seeing the doctor."

The urologist, Doctor F, examined Kyle and found a varicocele. The doctor explained that a varicocele is a mass of varicose veins in the testicle. The doctor told Kyle that medical science really does not know how a varicocele reduces sperm count, but he said that one theory hypothesizes that the accumulated blood in the varicose vein increases scrotal temperature, which in turn reduces sperm production. Kyle also had another sperm analysis done. The analysis showed that Kyle's sperm count was within the lower limits of normal, but the motility was greatly impaired. The doctor said that surgery helps improve sperm count and motility in about sixty to sixty-five percent of men. The surgery is performed under general anesthesia and consists of an incision in the groin; the internal spermatic vein is then tied.

Kyle and Sara were very nervous about surgery, but decided to go ahead with it. When Kyle was taken into surgery, Sara remembered thinking, "I was really worried for him. Somehow if it was something wrong with my body and it was my fault, it was okay. I could accept that. I didn't want it to be Kyle's problem. My sister and her husband didn't have children until seven years into their marriage because she had the infertility problem. So somehow, if it was all my fault it was okay. But Kyle's relatives are very prolific. Kyle's brother and sister-in-law could use three contraceptives at a time and still conceive. It just didn't seem fair it was happening to Kyle.

"When it was my problem I did things that helped me cope. I wrote, I would buy treats for myself, I would bury myself in work, and most importantly, I would share my pain with other people who understood. But Kyle really didn't have anyone to share his pain with besides me. That was really hard for me to see."

After surgery, another sperm analysis was done on Kyle. Neither the sperm count or motility had improved. Both Sara and Kyle were heartbroken. Sara said, "That was so depressing. All these years I've thought that the lab Kyle works in isn't good for him, because the chemicals he works with are so strong. Later we found out that the chemicals he works with are not supposed to affect motility. However, when he comes home and his breath smells so strongly of chemicals, you have to wonder."

At about this time the couple found out that Sara's physician, Doctor E, was no longer seeing patients. This fact, in combination with the outcome of Kyle's surgery, made them decide to stop the infertility treatments.

Five months after Kyle's surgery, the call came from their social worker about a boy named Josh. Sara remembered, "When we got the call, I thought, *We are going to adopt. Adoption must be what was meant for us.* We were told we had a week before Josh would come, and we went to the library and got every book on adoption we could get our hands on.

One of the phrases that jumped off the page at me was the statement that adoption does not fulfill the wants and needs of having a biological child. And my response was something like, 'What? It has to! That isn't fair. It *has* to meet my needs.' But Sara came to realize the statement was true: "While the adoption experience has been very fulfilling, it has not fulfilled that want or that desire for a baby. It hasn't fulfilled my desire to carry a baby in my body."

As they looked through Josh's file they were astounded to see that the beautiful three-year-old boy looked amazingly like his new father, Kyle. The couple was sickened to read about the abuse their son had taken. The report stated that Josh's stepfather had beaten him so severely that he had given Josh a skull fracture which ended up impairing his sight. Josh had been in and out of the hospital since birth for failure to thrive.

After Josh had been with Kyle and Sara for a short time, they took him to a speech therapist because of speech problems he was having. The specialist found that Josh had three anatomical abnormalities that were contributing to his speech difficulties. Sara remembered the rage she felt upon learning of his past, and said, "My anger and frustration over his treatment was immense. When he was a baby he couldn't even suck a bottle. Why wasn't this checked? It turned out that he had a short palate, and that was causing his inability to suck, and later his inability to speak normally. If Josh would have had surgery when he was a baby, he would not be having to endure years of speech therapy."

Within two weeks of the phone call about Josh, he was placed in their home. Sara and Kyle bonded with Josh immediately, although it took Josh a while to bond with his new parents. Since being taken from his birth mother and stepfather, Josh had been placed with a foster family while social services cleared the way for an adoption. Sara remembered, "The first two weeks was like living with a newborn, because he would wake up screaming in the night. He would cry, 'I had one mommy, then another mommy, and then another—I don't want any more mommies!'"

Sara had to fight for the right to take maternity leave to be with her new son. The leave was granted, however, and she took two full weeks off of work and then had afternoons off for the rest of the summer to spend with him. Sara was amazed at how many strong emotions she experienced when she held and rocked her new son. Having a child at home was very healing for both she and Kyle. Especially healing was the fact that Josh had been born a day after Sara's first miscarriage.

One fact that Kyle and Sara had been previously unaware of was that the adoption costs for their child with special needs were entirely covered by the state. They also found that there is funding available to pay for medical and educational needs, and they feel that this is an important fact for other couples considering adoption to know.

A number of changes took place after Josh came to live with Sara and Kyle. Sara stopped taking her basal body temperature and began to accept the possibility she might never become a biological mother. She said, "I had maternity clothes hanging in my closet, and it was part of my grieving process to let go of those. I gave them to someone who needed them." Although she was grieving for children she might never bear, she was rejoicing over her new son, Josh. After six months of having Josh, the couple contacted Social Services and asked for another child to be placed in their home.

To prepare for another child, the couple moved to another house. Sara remembered, "As we moved to the new house I came across a baby blanket that I had bought at some point, thinking it would go to my first baby. Josh asked, 'Mommy, is that what I was wrapped in when I was at the hospital?' He has always known he's adopted, but I think he forgot at that point. I said, 'No, honeybunch, but I sure wish it was.' I started to cry, and I realized that while I had bought this for my first baby, Josh was my first baby. So I gave the blanket to him. He is so proud of it. He has helped me lessen the pain of my infertility in so many ways."

When the social worker came to Sara and Kyle's house, Sara told the worker that she really wanted to adopt a girl. The social worker said that there were two girls in the system. One was a thirteen-year-old who had been sexually abused, and the other was a nine-year-old. The nine-year-old was in the process of being offered to another family for adoption. The social worker told the couple that the girl, Laura, was very smart, was a Baptist, played the piano, and was biracial. Sara said, "I can't begin to explain what hearing about her did to me. We are Baptist and love music, and she seemed to fit our family so well."

The couple began another ten-week-long adoption training, and at the first session, Sara and Kyle were given Laura's file to read. (The social worker explained that the other family had decided to let social services offer her to another family.) On their way home, Kyle and Sara discussed the fact that sometimes life can work out the way you hope it would.

"After that," Sara recalled, "the nightmare started. There had been a lot less information in Laura's file than we'd had in Josh's. We wondered why such an attractive and pleasant girl had been up for adoption, because the files didn't say. We thought of her as 'poor little Laura.' Later, we found out that Laura had been in and out of the system for seven years.

"When we brought her to our home for visits, she had no idea how to interact socially. We are a very social family, and we really wondered if we could change our lifestyle to meet her needs. The other thing we noticed was evidence of sexual problems; at nine years old, she was flirting with men. I don't think our marriage could have survived if we would have proceeded with the adoption. We had so much baggage from infertility, we decided we could not realistically meet her needs. It was a tough decision, but we declined the option to adopt her. Since then, we found out that her foster mom has adopted her."

Kyle and Sara questioned God about why they had to live with infertility and live through that experience with Laura. Sara said, "I questioned that a lot, and I finally realized that I didn't have to have a girl—that if I was ever to become pregnant, I wouldn't be disappointed if it was not a girl. Being pregnant by itself would be fine. I've come to believe that the experience was good, because Laura needed to find out how good she had it with her then-foster mother, social services needed to discover that her foster mother would make a good adoptive mother, and I needed it to realize I did not need to have a girl."

Coming down from such a heightened emotional experience was difficult for the couple, and it brought out feelings connected with their infertility once again. Both Kyle and Sara started to grieve their infertility more openly again. Sara said, "I feel the Scriptures really point to the importance of faith. One day I opened my Bible to this little verse. After I read the verse, a lot of my worries went away. It was like God was promising motherhood to me, because I just opened the Bible randomly. I didn't think we were going to adopt anymore and I looked at the verse and it said 'mother of children.' That was plural, and I have kept that phrase in my heart and mind."

Two months after the experience with Laura, Sara realized to her surprise that her menstrual cycles had become very regular. She began taking her temperature, and her charts showed regular cycles and a definite ovulatory pattern. Friends of the couple suggested that Sara see their reproductive endocrinologist, Doctor G. The couple was infertile, but with this doctor's help they had become pregnant.

Sara and Kyle discussed whether to proceed with more infertility treatments. Even though their past treatments had brought them so much grief, the pull to achieve a pregnancy was still very strong. Kyle said, "There is nothing in the world like holding a newborn baby. When I hold a newborn, there is such a deep desire within me to be able to hold my own baby."

Sara and Kyle went in for an appointment with the new doctor. He did a pelvic exam and a papsmear on Sara and told her that everything appeared normal.

The couple took an immediate liking to the doctor. Sara remembered, "He said that there would be days he was going to ask us to try and abstain from sex because of a particular test or treatment. But he said that if we wanted to have sex, we should. He gave us a license to enjoy our sexuality again; none of our other doctors even mentioned the possibility."

The doctor told them he wanted to do a few postcoital tests before scheduling any other type of treatments. Sara said, "We did several postcoital tests, and that was really frustrating. I ovulate late, and there would be hardly any mucus the day I would go in for the test. I would be dry as a bone on the thirteenth day, because I wouldn't ovulate till the fifteenth day. This procedure was really hurting our chances for conception, because we used the sperm up on the thirteenth day, and by the fifteenth there wasn't as much sperm as there could have been.

"As we continued with the tests, the doctor kept asking us if we were having intercourse, and we said we were. He told us he could not find any sperm in the mucus at all. At that point, Kyle had his count and motility rechecked. The count was excellent and the motility was sixty percent, which is good, but then it would drop off to one percent after a short amount of time."

Kyle and Sara grieved at the news. They once again felt they had no control over their reproductive life. With Sara ovulating on her own, they had begun to think there was a real possibility of producing a biological baby. To be teased into thinking of biological parenthood only to have their hopes dashed was crushing. Sara said, "I rejoice for others when they are pregnant. It is a gift from God. But I can still grieve my inability to have a baby. After hearing about Kyle's sperm, I received two phone calls within three hours from women who announced they were pregnant. Two announcements in three hours is a little much."

Sara tried to put the prognosis into perspective, to go on with her life as normally as possible. But she reached a point when she really needed to share her grief with someone. Sara said, "A few months earlier, my sister-in-law had shared the news of her latest pregnancy with us early on. We had been trying to start a better relationship, so I thought I'd step out on a limb and share with her the news about Kyle's sperm. Her reaction was, 'Just let me send my husband over there, and he'll help you out.' She was joking, but it was cruel. I felt totally shattered that day."

A month later, Sara and Kyle were told they were getting close to having another child placed with them, so they decided to put a hold on any further infertility treatments. One evening they arrived home to find a message on their answering machine from their social worker. The message instructed them to call the social worker at home to find out about a possible child to be placed. They called that evening and found out that there was a little boy named R.J. who was available. The worker told them R.J. was in a good foster home, he had a speech delay, and had hearing problems as an infant which had apparently now cleared up. She told the couple they could pick his file up at the office if they wanted to.

They were scheduled to leave for vacation the next day, but on the way Kyle and Sara picked up R.J.'s file. Sara recalled, "I read Kyle the information on our way to Wisconsin. Reading the file out loud was pretty emotional because of the severe neglect R.J. had experienced. The report stated that his birth mom bragged to people that she was drinking a six pack a day when she was pregnant with R.J. (I had heard that alcoholics disclose only about one third of the amount they actually drink, so I imagined she could have actually been drinking a twelve pack or more.) R.J. had been locked in one room for a year of his life and been let out only a few times a day. His birth mom had six other children. Four of the older children were living with their birth dad. It was very hard to read about his life and know that he had brothers and sisters out there."

As part of the adoption process, prospective parents make a book about themselves for the child to read. It helps the child get used to the fact that he or she will have a new family. Sara said, "We made a book for R.J. that told him all about us, and then we made an appointment to see him the next week. When we got there, R.J.'s social worker handed us the book and told us he hadn't seen it yet. The foster family R.J. had been placed with had not prepared R.J. for adoption at all.

"When we got there I asked to see R.J.'s room. I was told he didn't have one. The foster family had been waiting to adopt a newborn baby, and had redone R.J.'s room to make it into a nursery. R.J. did not have a room, or a bed to sleep on, and he didn't even have a dresser drawer he could call his own. He had been sleeping on the floor." Not only was the couple angered by R.J.'s treatment, they were furious when the social worker told them he was not yet legally free for adoption. Social Services was still advertising in the newspaper to try to locate R.J.'s birth mother. The case-worker told the couple they would need to become foster parents first, and when parental rights were severed they could adopt R.J.

By that point, however, the couple felt committed to keeping R.J. This little boy had been tossed around so much, and they did not want to contribute to the process. Of the adoption, Kyle said, "R.J.'s adoption has not been like Josh's. We have had wonderful times with R.J., but they have been very few. He has severe attachment problems, and continually tests us."

Sara felt that R.J.'s foster dad had never released R.J. to love his new family. She said, "His foster parents were 'fost-adopt' parents. That is, they could elect to adopt R.J. once he was available. His foster mom chose not to adopt R.J., but the foster dad, Randy, wanted to. This has been a continuing problem, because he hasn't let go of R.J. He did not show up for the November farewell ceremony for R.J., but in December, his foster parents wanted to have an overnight farewell party. They had had him for two years and said they wanted to be him with him for one last time. We agreed, and Randy came to get R.J. When he came, R.J. called him 'daddy,' and Randy did not correct him. Randy told R.J. to give me a hug—Randy didn't refer to me as 'mom', which is a necessary part of attachment. When R.J. refused, Randy said, 'If you don't give Sara a hug, you will have to stay here.' I was just livid! I said, 'Like that would be an awful thing.'"

After R.J. had visited his foster parents, attachment seemed like it would never happen. Sara and Kyle tried very hard to show affection to R.J. and help the attachment process. They referred to him as "my R.J." and tried to give him control and ownership when possible. Sara recalled, "The joy on R.J.'s face when he got to put his clothes in his drawer and got to sleep on his Mickey Mouse sheets in his own bed was wonderful to see."

Before adopting R.J., Sara had scheduled three infertility procedures to be done in December. She had an x-ray done on her tubes and uterus and a biopsy of the lining of her womb, but she postponed the diagnostic laparoscopy until R.J. became more comfortable in their home. Sara recalled, "I really was still interested in pursuing infertility treatments. The first time they checked the lining of my womb, the results said that it was not preparing for implantation, but the second test said it was. That made me wonder if my hormones weren't at a consistent level. The doctor told me that because I had had problems with implantation in the past, I would be on progesterone to keep the pregnancy viable if one occurred. They also injected dye into the tubes, and I had thoroughly dreaded that. My sister had had that done in a doctor's office and said it was the most painful thing she had ever gone through. But my doctor did the procedure differently than hers had. He put a clamp on my cervix, and the dye was injected. It was not painful at all; I kept waiting for the pain to get worse, and it didn't. I got to see the dye go through the tubes on the x-ray. It flowed out of the left tube fine, but took longer to spill through the right tube. Seeing the dye go through the tubes was amazing. I sat up and I wanted to hug my doctor when he said the tubes looked good. He said he felt that if Kyle's sperm was washed and then I was artificially inseminated, the chances for a pregnancy would be improved, but informed me that I would have to have a laparoscopy first." Sara and Kyle were thrilled with the news. They knew if the laparoscopy turned out well, a biological child might be a possibility again.

Soon after these medical procedures were done, they got the news that R.J. was now legally free for adoption. Kyle said, "Life with R.J. had been very up and down. There were a couple of days in January when we very seriously considered taking him back."

Sara put off scheduling the laparoscopy because she felt it was important to focus on trying to help R.J. adjust to his new family. After a few months, Sara decided it was time to resume infertility treatments. She called the head nurse at the doctor's office and said she was interested in finding a time to have a laparoscopy done. The nurse told Sara to send in her basal body temperature graphs, but Sara told the nurse that she had not kept any charts since November. The nurse then informed Sara that the doctor would need at least one cycle charted. Sara remembered, "I took my temperature every day that month and called to make the appointment. The nurse told me that my doctor was going to be on vacation the day I needed to have surgery, so I had to wait yet another month to get it done."

While waiting for the day of the surgery to arrive, Sara experienced three events that made waiting very difficult. The first event was Mother's Day. Sara remembered, "Before Josh, Mother's Day was very hard for me. I would not go to church because I could not handle the emotional impact of it. Having Josh as my son changed that, but it was weird because on that Mother's Day I had a hard time at church. I felt strange standing when they asked all mothers in the congregation to stand. I had not felt that way the past few years, but this year was hard for me because I had not biologically produced a child. That had been weighing on my mind since we started our infertility treatments again. After the service I went home and cried. I called my sister and she came over to grieve with me."

The previous December, Sara had hired a woman at the company where she worked. The woman had asked Sara when she could get pregnant and still be covered by insurance, and Sara had told her that if she got pregnant after June first, insurance would be in effect. In the middle of June, the woman reported to Sara that she had gotten pregnant June second. Sara said, "As she told me, I kept thinking what a luxury that was. Her announcement brought back my bitterness and frustration towards Josh's and R.J.'s birth moms, who had the ability to become pregnant again and again. What my boys went through, no children should ever have to go through. But the law really protects birth moms. R.J.'s birth mom could have kids even though she drank a six pack a day. She could have kids even in jail. For me, dealing with that anger is a very tough issue."

Another event that cut Sara very deeply in June was the attitude of her parents when they visited from Japan. Sarah recalled, "My parents had come to visit, and the first thing out of their mouths as we met them was a story about their new granddaughter, who, incidentally, was named after my mother. Here she is excited about this new granddaughter, and I'm thinking, *You have a new grandson you haven't met. Why aren't you excited about him? He counts, too.*"

Sara made the appointment for the surgery in July. She said, "I was amazed at how calm I was the week of the surgery. The day before the laparoscopy, my doctor had me come in for a pre-surgery checkup. He asked me if I did monthly self-checks on my breasts, and I said no. He examined the first breast and upon checking the other one, I said, 'Ooh, that hurts.' He responded, 'It should—it's a lump.'

"I just started to freak out. I wanted to scream at him. My mind started racing in every direction. I know there are many women who have had lumps removed; the strange side of it was that I already had a whammy against me because I couldn't produce children. I thought that if I had to have a breast removed because of cancer, I didn't know how I would cope."

The doctor told her he would still do the laparoscopy the next day, but would not do any further infertility treatments until the lump was removed by a surgeon. He went on to tell Sara that he wanted her to cycle before making an appointment with a surgeon, because there was a chance the lump could disappear as the cycle started. Sara said, "Thinking about it now, I believe God directed this. I never did exams, and the doctor just happened to do one. The night before the pre-surgery check I'd had an odd feeling, and I called a woman to see if she would teach Sunday school for me so I could recover during the weekend. I asked her what she was doing the next day, and she said she was going to the same town that my doctor's appointment was at. So we decided to go together. I was glad she was there for support, because Kyle had been unable to come with me. I came out of the office crying, and we left right away."

After the laparoscopy the doctor had told Sara that her fallopian tubes had flipped over on the ovaries, which had resulted in some scar tissue. He had recommended superovulation cycles for four months—Sara would take medication to stimulate her ovaries into making as many as eggs as possible. Using this procedure in tandem with artificial insemination, the doctor was hopeful that at least one egg would be able to find its way into the tube to be fertilized. He had gone on to say that most women did not usually get pregnant during the first cycle, but if there was not a pregnancy after four cycles, the chance of a pregnancy occurring with that form of treatment was unlikely. Finally, the doctor told Sara and Kyle that the cost per cycle for superovulation would be approximately two thousand dollars.

At the time this chapter is written, Sara and Kyle have not started the superovulation cycles. Sara said, "Before the last surgery, Kyle and I had decided that we would try twelve cycles of artificial insemination. Now, with this treatment, we only have four months to try to achieve a pregnancy. Four cycles seems so limiting. I have mixed feelings about the superovulation cycles. They will cost two thousand dollars for one cycle. We really haven't resolved whether or not we will do it; it's hard to spend eight thousand dollars with no guarantee. We could adopt a newborn for that much money.

"We are in the process of wondering if our desires are selfish or misdirected. The doctor keeps telling me that if I get this straightened out I have ten years of childbearing left. In a few more years we will be better able to afford this procedure, but I don't want to be thirty-five and have my biological clock ticking and wonder why we didn't do the procedure before. We have a good relationship with the bank, and I know we could ask for a baby loan if we had to."

Sara will wait until her cycle starts to determine if the lump is still there. If it is, she will need to have the lump removed and biopsied. If the lump is benign, Sara and Kyle will try to conceive a baby in the month prior to the superovulation cycles naturally, by using Robitussin expectorant and a douche. They hope that the cough syrup and the douche will make the cervical mucus thinner, so sperm can move through it. Sara said, "We had friends who were infertile for five years and tried the Robitussin and the douche and got pregnant the first month. Another thing that might help is the fact that about four months ago, Kyle's lab had a hood installed to ventilate the work area. Since then, the volume of his semen seems to have increased. We hope that we can create a miracle."

Four days after the laparoscopy, Sara and Kyle took R.J. to see a developmental specialist. He gave the couple some discouraging news about R.J.'s development. According to this doctor, it is a miracle R.J. is as normal as he is for all the abuse and neglect he suffered. Physically, R.J. is developing on schedule. Emotionally, socially, and cognitively, however, R.J. is still trying to catch up to his peers. R.J. has auditory memory loss, is having severe attachment problems, and has problems knowing how to interact in large groups. The doctor said R.J. was treatable, but that preventive services needed to start immediately, and could not wait until he was in elementary school, as previously thought.

Sara and Kyle came home emotionally shell shocked. To find out about a lump in Sara's breast, the expense of the recommended infertility procedure, and the severity of R.J.'s developmental problems in less than a week's time was understandably traumatic for the couple. They wondered how they could make even one decision when there were so many factors to sort through. But they sat down and discussed what their options were. Both Kyle and Sara said that their decisions changed from moment to moment, which is why they have decided to bring their friends into their decision making.

The couple feels that they no longer can carry the emotional baggage of infertility alone. Sara said, "We are having a gathering in our home next week for a time of healing prayer. We are sending a letter to family we know can't come and to six couples we are close to. Infertility has been a taboo subject, and we have decided after years of struggle that it will not be so taboo with our friends any longer. We are taking a plunge, and it is so scary. But to make a good decision we think we need other people's support—up until this point we pretty much have faced our infertility alone. I think it will be very healing for us."

As Sara and Kyle prepared for their night of prayer, Sara reflected on the children that are already in their lives. She said, "Infertility is not the big ugly monster it was before adoption. The nurturing and the love are there even though the feelings of frustration I have over not being able to produce a child are increased by seeing people who can easily conceive children, only to torment them. At times my bitterness towards my sons' birth moms is overwhelming, but there is a part of me that thanks them for not having abortions, so we could have the boys.

"Infertility is a lack of control, and adoption brings control back into your life. No matter the outcome of our infertility, the boys I have now are our sons, and no one can ever take that from us. Yet, I also know that our longing for a baby is still there, and no one can ever take that away from us either."

4

How much expense is too much in the process of trying to conceive a child? How much time and effort should we put into creating a life? Are new technologies, such as the use of donor sperm, unethical or immoral? Why are we infertile? What is God's plan for us as parents? Will we ever feel happy or content with our lives again? These are some of the questions Lisa and Bill have struggled with for the past nine years. They haven't found the answers and their pain has not diminished, but they have not given up hope.

When Lisa and Bill started dating, friends and family remarked that they had a storybook romance. As individuals, both were vibrant, energetic people. When together, their personal energies melded and resulted in an incredibly strong and committed marriage. Together they felt there was nothing they could not accomplish.

Both felt a strong respect for family. Lisa and Bill truly loved children and were looking forward to the time when their love would produce their own. Lisa had loved babies from the time she was a child. Anytime there was a baby around, she would ask to hold and cuddle it. Many times the baby would have to be taken away from her, because she did not want to give it up. Yet oddly enough, as a young child Lisa felt that she would have difficulty having children, although she also felt that twins were in her future. Where these feelings sprang from has eluded Lisa, but they have always been very strong impressions.

Prior to their marriage, Bill would ask Lisa how many children she wanted. She remembered saying, "Two for sure, and maybe three." Bill would then say, "Or four, five, or six?" They would then laugh and feel enveloped in the security of their fertility. Lisa interpreted the statements as her husband's desire for a large family. Bill, on the other hand, recalled this as flirtatious banter. He said, "I was just kidding around. I didn't know that after we got married we would have problems with infertility. My words have come back to haunt me."

Lisa and Bill were married in February of 1984, and Lisa began taking birth control pills. A few months later, she asked Bill if he would mind if she discontinued the pills. They discussed the issue, and both agreed that a pregnancy would be a wonderful event in their lives. Lisa said, "Although I didn't expect to get pregnant the first month, I did expect to be pregnant relatively soon. I had a friend who was pregnant then, and I just knew we were going to have our babies at the same time. Then I thought, well, maybe they'll be a month apart, or two months apart, and I'd keep going on like that."

The pregnancy that Lisa had hoped for did not happen. What was growing inside Lisa was not a baby, but a feeling of dread. With each passing month Lisa was reintroduced to the cycle of grief that infertile women know intimately.

This was an incredibly difficult time for Lisa, and there was not a good support system available to her. Because Bill was in the military, they were living in a different state than her friends and family. Lisa was in a new town, with few friends to confide in, secretly fearing that her most treasured dream of becoming a mother was, indeed, only a dream. She eventually confided in an acquaintance and was told to chart her basal body temperature before making an appointment with a gynecologist. Lisa took her temperature for six months, hoping to pinpoint ovulation and time intercourse for her most fertile period. She methodically recorded each day's temperature and soon had a stack of monthly charts that indicated she was ovulating regularly. Yet month after month, the charts also indicated she was not pregnant. They were, to her, a written record of her failure.

After six months, Lisa made an appointment with a gynecologist, Doctor A. He did an endometrial biopsy which indicated that Lisa was not ovulating. The test, now commonly thought to be an outdated evaluation procedure, is an indirect way to determine if and when a woman ovulates. The procedure involves taking a bit of endometrial tissue from the woman in the second half of her cycle and examining it under a microscope.

Lisa also had a hysterosalpinogram—an x-ray of her uterus and tubes. The x-ray procedure consists of having an opaque liquid injected into the cervix. An x-ray is then taken to see if the liquid runs through the fallopian tubes freely. The doctor said her tubes appeared to be clear. He recommended another endometrial biopsy and the fertility drug Clomid.

The doctor also ran a semen analysis on Bill. He indicated that the results were on the low range of normal. Lisa remembered, "I know that he told us the count was low, but what I had in my mind was that it was normal. I pushed it out of my mind and was not concerned about it. But as we went through infertility treatments, every semen analysis that came back had 'abnormal' on it. I don't know if it was my way of protecting the male ego or what, but I didn't discuss it with him. I know that it is harder for the man, and I think I wanted it to be my problem rather than Bill's. I wanted to protect him from that."

Before Lisa could continue treatment with Doctor A, she and Bill moved back to their home state. She began to see another gynecologist, Doctor B, and told her of the previous doctor's findings. This doctor put Lisa on Clomid, and soon after she ovulated, Lisa suspected a pregnancy. Lisa said, "It was right before Mother's Day, and we had been trying to have a baby for about two years. I told Bill I wanted to go in and have a pregnancy test done. I wanted to be able to tell the news of the pregnancy to our moms on Mother's Day. He said, 'Don't do it. When the tests come back negative you are going to be a bitch for the weekend. I don't want you to do it.' I didn't listen to him. I went in, and the pregnancy test came back positive. I can still remember—you'd think I'd be so excited—but I just sat there and said, 'really?'"

Bill and Lisa went to his mother's house and broke their news. Everyone was thrilled for the couple. That evening, Lisa started spotting. She had no idea what the spotting meant. She was unsure if it was normal or if it was signaling the death of her baby. Not wanting to upset Bill's family, she did not tell them of her bleeding.

The next day, her in-laws kept asking her to tell other family members her good news. Lisa remembered, "I told them the news, but it was really hard, because I wasn't excited about it anymore. I thought I would have to go back and tell them I wasn't pregnant any longer. I didn't want to tell them without knowing what was going on."

Bill and Lisa went home after the weekend, and she called her doctor. She told Lisa to take it easy and to try and rest. But as the bleeding continued, her anxiety rose, and she finally told her doctor that she had to know what was going on.

At this point, Lisa was unsure of what to think. Was this a miscarriage or a part of her pregnancy? Her doctor did an ultrasound and found the gestational sac, but was unable at that point to find the heartbeat. She sent Lisa to the hospital, where they had a highly sensitive ultrasound machine. The baby's heartbeat was located. The reason for the bleeding was unknown, but Lisa decided to take the cautious route. She went on complete bed rest for the first trimester to try to improve the chances of keeping the pregnancy viable.

Within minutes of beginning the second ultrasound, Lisa had gone from feeling incredible fear to experiencing overwhelming joy. To spend three months in bed to assure her baby's health was an act of love that she relished. Lisa said, "It kills me now to hear what people say when there seems to be a problem during pregnancy. A friend of my mom was pregnant with twins, and she miscarried one of them, but she was still carrying the other. But her mother told her that bleeding is a sign the baby is abnormal. So the pregnant woman worked herself to death to try to get the baby to spontaneously abort, and it did. I don't know how people can say those things."

After the first trimester the pregnancy was uneventful, but during the later stages, Bill was transferred to another state. He told Lisa that it would be best if she stayed with her parents. He was concerned about the amount of time he would be away from home and felt that she needed to be with people to help and support her during the pregnancy. This was a difficult decision to make, but eventually both partners decided it was for the best. Lisa and Bill passed the last few weeks of the pregnancy thinking of each other and wondering what their new baby would be like.

After weeks of anxious waiting, Lisa began labor. She learned from her doctor that the baby's heart rate was dropping during each contraction, and although this was not a desperate cause for alarm, it certainly concerned Lisa. When her son was born, he had the cord wrapped around his neck and was holding onto it with his hand. The drop in heart rate was attributed to Matt squeezing the cord as he made his way into the world. Lisa chuckled to herself as she held her son in her arms. Not only was he not abnormal, as some might have suggested, he was a plucky little fighter, a son well worth waiting for.

Bill remembered his son's birth: "Being at the birth was pretty special for me. At the time, I didn't realize just how special it was. We were both there together looking at the child that we had made."

Matt was about six weeks old before Bill and Lisa were once again reunited. Bill had been transferred again, and they moved shortly thereafter to yet another state. They had found a nice house and begun to settle into their new home and their new life when Bill brought up the idea of trying to have another baby. Lisa remembered, "I was shocked; I told him I just couldn't. He and his sister are thirteen months apart, and he just thought it was a great way to grow up. He had such fond memories of his childhood, yet I came from a family with five kids who were born in six years. I hate to say it, but what I remember is my mom always being frazzled and never having enough time, and I didn't want that. Not that I had a bad childhood, because I didn't. But I wanted the best for my child, and I thought it would be better if there was a bigger space between the children. I kept putting him off, and feeling guilty about it."

Bill said, "I wanted another child after Matt was born. I don't know—it's hard to say what would have happened if we'd tried for another child right away. But I didn't force the issue since she was the one who would have to carry the child. It's hard to not think about what might have happened, though."

When Matt was a year old, Bill and Lisa moved back to their home state. During the move Lisa lost the applicator for the contraceptive foam they were using and decided at that point to let nature take its course. Lisa did not really want a pregnancy, though, and every time she got her period she was silently thankful. A few months later, however, Lisa began to wonder if she was pregnant. She was exhausted, had a tender stomach, and felt very lethargic. Lisa went to the doctor and found out that she and Matt both had contracted a virus from drinking tainted water. She remembered telling the doctor that she was surprised to feel a bit disappointed that she was not pregnant. Lisa said, "So maybe from there I started wanting to be pregnant more, and yet the timing wasn't right. It wasn't my idea of how I wanted the timing. I still wanted my children farther apart, but I think something clicked on in me—a fear. Even though it was maybe something I wouldn't have wanted right then, I began to be afraid that I wouldn't be be able to have another child. So the process started again."

Six months later, Lisa contacted her family practitioner, Doctor C. She told him of her desire for a pregnancy, and of her background with Clomid. Lisa asked him if he could prescribe Clomid, or if she would need to be seen by an obstetrician again. The doctor said he would talk to her previous obstetrician and get her advice. A week later he called Lisa and told her that her previous obstetrician would like to see her. She remembered thinking, *That's fine.* "I knew that you really should have an exam to make sure your ovaries aren't enlarged before you start taking Clomid, so I made the appointment, but she didn't even examine me. She informed me that she would work with me, reviewed my medical charts with me, wrote out a prescription for Clomid, and left. I thought maybe she just wanted to charge me for the office visit, but as far as I was concerned she could have charged me over the phone and saved me the time, because my time is worth more than that." What many doctors seem to be unaware of is the incredible amount of tension and anxiety that surround an office visit. Infertility is difficult enough to survive without adding the stress of an unnecessary trip to the doctor.

Lisa was given the prescription for six months of Clomid, but was not given any guidance about what she could expect. Many clinics do a Clomid check on women after a new cycle begins to check for ovarian cysts, as well as to give the patient a chance to ask the medical questions she has. Lisa remembered, "There I was, floundering without any doctor care, and just not knowing. Of course, I could not talk to her—only her nurse. I called her nurse to try and get some answers. Whether I asked to see the doctor or just asked questions of her, she seemed really put out." The nurse did ask if Lisa was ovulating, and Lisa answered yes. After six months, Lisa called the nurse again. Lisa remembered the nurse seemed annoyed. The nurse told her, "If you really want I could make an appointment for you to come up and see the doctor."

When Lisa went to the clinic, she was informed that her doctor was out on a delivery. Furthermore, Lisa was told she would not be in after that for two weeks because she was going on vacation. At this point, Lisa lost her patience with the medical staff. After explaining her irritation with them for not cancelling her appointment before she made the trip, she asked to see another doctor.

The next day she was seen by another doctor, Doctor D, who told her that she had a cyst the size of a tennis ball on her ovary. Lisa said, "That frightened me to the bone, because I have a sister who a year before that had lost one of her tubes and her ovary because of a big cyst on her ovary that had flipped and cut circulation off to the tube. That was all I could think about, that at any minute this thing was going to flip and I would lose half of my chances for getting pregnant."

Lisa was scheduled for a cystectomy via laparoscopy two days later. After the surgery the doctor told Lisa that the tubes looked good, and that the cyst had been removed. He advised her to try and achieve a pregnancy without Clomid for three cycles. He said he felt sure she would get pregnant within this time frame.

Lisa felt that finally she was making progress, and started to genuinely hope for a pregnancy. Her relief was short-lived, however, because she found out that her insurance company refused to pay for her surgery because it did not have the operative report. After many delays between the clinic and insurance company, Lisa picked up a copy of the report and sent it to the insurance company herself. Before sending it, however, she read the report. It said that during the laparoscopy, the doctor had tried to inject methane blue dye through the cervix, but the tenaculum, or clamp, fell off, and it was impossible. Lisa remembered feeling very angry with the doctor. She said, "He told me that everything was fine and he didn't even have a chance to see." Lisa was totally disenchanted by the apparent deception and seeming negligence of the doctors she had worked with. It was at this time that she made an appointment with a highly-regarded reproductive endocrinologist, Doctor E, hoping for some straightforward answers.

The catch was that the earliest the doctor could see Lisa was five months later. Waiting long periods of time between infertility treatments can ravage the infertile person's feelings of hope and control. Lisa believes she survived the rough moments by talking to her best friend, another woman struggling with infertility. Lisa and her friend Alisha talked often of the feelings infertility evoked.

But sometimes, even women who share infertility inadvertently hurt each other. Lisa remembered, "One day I was feeling particularly low, and I went to talk to Alisha. I was talking about my desire for another child, and she said to me, 'Lisa, don't take this the wrong way, but why do you want another baby? You have a child already—you're very fortunate. Why do you have to have another?' At that point I just shut up. I felt I couldn't talk to her about my struggles anymore, that I must be putting too much pressure on her. I had one child, while she had none. I felt guilty for having a child, and she did not realize that having a child does not make the desire for another one any less."

Lisa attempted to avoid talking about her infertility to Alisha, but one day she realized how much she needed Alisha's support. Lisa confronted Alisha and said, "Alisha, I was really bothered by what you said. When you asked me why Matt wasn't enough, did you think I'm depriving him in my attempts to have another baby?" When Alisha said no, Lisa asked what her comment had meant. Alisha responded, "Just what I said. I think you are fortunate to have one child and should keep that in mind." Lisa then replied, "Alisha, you're planning a trip to Italy, and you appreciate travelling, right?" When Alisha nodded, Lisa went on to say, "If you appreciated trips you've taken, why do you want to take another one? By your reasoning, it must mean you don't appreciate what you have. If you want to go on another trip, you can't have appreciated the others." It was at that point that Alisha said, "I think I understand now."

What many people (including many infertile people without children) don't realize is that having one child does not mean that the couple's needs have been met. The couple loves their child and acknowledges how fortunate they are to have a child, but that does not mean that the desire for another child goes away. A couple can truly love their first, and wanting another child is completely normal. Lisa explained, "I hate having to feel guilty for wanting another child. I hate having to defend why I have this desire. What people don't know is that even if a baby comes into a family, the desire for another one is there. Also present is grief. Infertility is grieving the loss of normalcy. I am made to feel abnormal for wanting my second child, while fertile people can want many children without being questioned about their feelings."

The time for Lisa's appointment finally arrived. She was impressed by the endocrinologist's thoroughness and knowledge. After one pelvic exam he told her that her left side was fuller than her right side, that her uterus was pulling off to the right, and that she probably had endometriosis. He scheduled Lisa for yet another laparoscopy.

The laparoscopy is usually scheduled at midcycle or a few days before. Due to scheduling problems, however, they had to wait until a few days after Lisa's midcycle. She was told to use birth control during this time to make sure a pregnancy would not occur. Lisa laughed at the notion of using birth control; to think that a pregnancy would result within a month after years of trying was ludicrous.

Her period was on time, and then, two weeks later, she started bleeding. Because nothing like this had ever happened to her, she became frightened and called her new doctor. He told Lisa there was a possibility she had been pregnant and had spontaneously miscarried. Lisa said, "I was surprised at the depth of how that hit me, because I had a normal period, not expecting anything. Yet once he told me there was a possibility, that baby was just as alive to me as if I had carried it full term."

Both a laparoscopy and a D & C were done shortly thereafter. The doctor found that both ovaries were enlarged, and discovered some tissue that could be endometriosis. He advised Lisa to have a laparotomy so he could do a further diagnosis. She was told that a laparotomy would require an incision in the abdomen and a recovery period both at the hospital and at home.

At this point in her medical experiences, Lisa was very wary of yet another procedure. She soon found out that this surgery would be counted among the bad experiences. She was advised to be at the hospital at six a.m. the day of her surgery. Lisa checked in and waited for over an hour for her name to be called. Finally, a nurse called her name and asked how long she had been there. The nurse had not realized that Lisa was present because there had been a mix-up at the front desk. She was told that surgery would have to take place immediately, and that they would need to hurry to get her ready. Lisa remembered, "They gave me an enema, and I was in the bathroom for only a couple of minutes before they started asking me to come out because there was a lab technician there to draw my blood. And I'm like, 'Give me a break! Just give me some time to sit on this toilet.' I mean, I was already nervous. They give you this enema for a reason, and I wanted to get cleaned out so there wouldn't be any embarrassing situations once I got into surgery. They told me that if I came out, they would let me sit on the toilet again after they took the blood. Then they told me that the anesthetist was there, and that I needed to come out and talk with him. I was just in tears. When they came in to get me, they probably thought I was some whacko lady.

"This surgery was more stressful to me than the laparoscopy. I mean, I had a small child at home, and here they are rushing me through this. The doctor came in to talk to me and his nurse held my hand as they walked me down the corridor. I still had tears running down my face as they administered the anesthesia." Lisa's recovery took much longer than what is normally expected. She feels that her treatment at the hospital prior to surgery and the emotions and tension it evoked greatly influenced her recovery time.

Lisa's doctor discussed the results of the diagnostic laparotomy with her. He told her that her uterus was attached to the right ovary with scar tissue, that both tubes had scar tissue, with one being one hundred percent blocked and the other having only a minute opening, and that the opening to the uterus was larger than normal. He went on to tell her that he had removed ten cysts from her ovaries. According to the doctor, it had been rather miraculous that she had gotten pregnant with her first child.

Lisa could not believe the news. This information was at odds with all she had heard previously from other doctors. She remembered thinking, "I knew I had a miracle at home, but I did not realize how much of a miracle he was. That egg should have never gotten through that small hole, and I should never have been able to carry him to full term. I guess that is one thing that has come out of my infertility: the ability to appreciate all that I have. I am very thankful for that, and I think that it makes me a better mother."

In spite of what the doctor had found, Lisa and Bill felt that the surgery was going to be the difference—that in a few short months they would know that God had granted them another miracle. Four months passed without a pregnancy, however, and Bill was advised to have another semen analysis done. The results stated that his ejaculate was twice that of a normal man's, and diluted the concentration of the sperm. The doctor advised him to do a split ejaculate. The idea was that the sperm would be concentrated in the first part of the ejaculate, and would be less likely to have abnormalities. Lisa and Bill were told that gathering a split ejaculate and using artificial insemination would probably solve their fertility problems. Lisa remembered Bill saying, "I'm supposed to get half in this cup and half in the other? How am I going to do that?" Fortunately, Bill and Lisa somehow managed to view the situation with humor. Fertile couples have the luxury of having sex to produce a baby. Infertile couples have to go through many varied and humiliating procedures to try to produce a child.

Infertile couples are constantly restructuring their views on what they will do in order to conceive a baby. When a couple works together and sees humor in the situation, stress is reduced. Despite the mounting problems caused by their infertility, Lisa and Bill tried to find whatever shreds of humor existed in their situation.

Lisa had two cycles of artificial insemination which did not result in a pregnancy. She asked her endocrinologist if she could go back on the fertility drug, Clomid. He told her it was probably just a fluke that she had gotten pregnant while using the drug. Lisa remembered, "I told him it probably was more of a fluke than anything else, but I would feel better—I would feel like I was doing everything I could." The doctor acquiesced to her request, telling her that it wouldn't hurt her chances.

Lisa had been on Clomid for four months when her doctor abruptly quit his practice because of health concerns. Lisa was upset about her doctor leaving his practice, but she had been having difficulty with scheduling problems. Because of the doctor's health, he had cut back to being in his office only four days out of the month. Lisa had had to juggle the doctor's schedule, her ovulation day, and her husband's work schedule. This was virtually impossible, because her husband was out of town for fifteen to sixteen days of the month. They would get the timing close, but never exact. The stress this produced for Lisa and Bill was incredible, so as they were faced with changing doctors once again, it was at the same time a nerve wracking experience and a relief.

By this point, Lisa and Bill had gone through so much stress that they wondered if their marriage would ever be the same. They were on a constant roller coaster of stress and disappointment. There were many days when Lisa forced herself to get out of bed and get on with the day.

One day, Lisa's sister Becky came to see her. She had an offer: Becky told Lisa that she and her husband had noticed the emotional stress that infertility was causing the couple and that Becky and her husband Dave had discussed Lisa and Bill's infertility at length. Becky offered to be the couple's surrogate mother.

This was not a decision that was lightly researched or easily decided upon. Becky and her husband had even seen a lawyer to discuss legal issues involving a surrogacy. Lisa remembered thinking that she knew her sister could handle the emotional impact of a surrogacy, but she was unsure whether she would be able to. Lisa was very close to Becky, and the thought of avoiding her sister because of the fear that Becky might become attached to the baby was much too painful for Lisa to consider. Lisa feels that her sister offered the most sincere, most beautiful gift of love that anyone has ever given her. But it was a gift she couldn't accept.

Lisa knew she needed to continue to try to work toward a biological pregnancy. She asked the endocrinologist's head nurse for a referral. (Lisa remembered wondering how in the world she was supposed to choose from all the doctors available.) The nurse told her there was another reproductive endocrinologist, Doctor F, in town, but she did not know much about his practice. She told Lisa that the only thing she did know was that he did not have as many patients as the doctor she had worked for. She then recommended Doctor G, who was not a reproductive endocrinologist, but who was doing a lot of work in the infertility field. Lisa made an appointment to see him the next month.

To change to yet another doctor, one whom she had never met, was one more emotional setback for Lisa. For an infertile couple, a sense of control is vital to stay sane, and when you have to keep juggling doctors, new treatments, and new philosophies, control is lost. Lisa went in to see the doctor feeling very anxious. She remembered, "He told me that I had seen a lot of doctors, and that we needed to wipe the slate clean and start again. By this time I had been trying to conceive for three years after giving birth to my son, and there had been two years prior to his conception. In total, I'd had five years of infertility workups, many surgeries, a wealth of hope, and a bunch of medical dead ends. All of these I was supposed to banish. They weren't being counted." Lisa couldn't believe what he was asking of her; the doctor's approach to infertility made her extremely uncomfortable, but she wondered if she left his care, where else would she go?

The doctor did a PK test on Lisa to evaluate whether Bill's sperm was able to move freely within her cervical mucus, and performed another endometrial biopsy. He found there was not a lot of sperm in the mucus and advised Lisa and Bill to resume artificially inseminated cycles using the split ejaculate. He also ordered three more semen analyses to check on the sperm.

After two cycles of artificial insemination he advised Bill to see a urologist. The urologist, Doctor H, examined Bill and told him he had a varicocele—a varicose vein of the testicle. Many urologists believe that surgery can improve both pregnancy rates and sperm count. This was an incredibly difficult decision for Bill, as he is a pilot, and the surgery would mean he would not be able to fly for a significant portion of a month.

At the same time, Bill had an annual physical which was done by his employer's doctors. The doctors reported that Bill had an enlarged spleen, and his employers would not let him fly until it was taken care of. Bill went to an oncologist, Doctor I, who informed him there was no cause for concern over the enlarged spleen. Tests had ruled out cancer and leukemia. There was a long list of medical maladies that were also tested for, and none of those had caused the spleen enlargement. However, the oncologist did tell him that he had the mono antibody in his blood, and that it could be mononucleosis. If it was mononucleosis, it could take up to three months for the swelling in the spleen to go down. In conclusion, the doctor told Bill he could live normally with his spleen in its current condition. His employers, however, told him that unless something was done, he would still not be able to fly. (The reason for this was that because of the G forces he experienced when he flew, Bill had to wear a G suit. The G suit inflates and puts pressure on the body, and with an enlarged spleen, this could be dangerous.)

Because flying was such a joy for Bill, he could not envision giving it up. After a long discussion, he and Lisa decided they would go to a regional medical center for a second opinion. Bill also wanted to see a urologist while he was there, because he felt that if he was going to have one surgery (his employer's physician suggested surgery on his spleen) that would keep him from work, he might as well get both surgeries over at the same time.

But a new urologist, Doctor J, did an ultrasound on Bill's testicles and informed him that there was no varicocele present. Bill and Lisa were shocked at the news and said, "But they told us there was a varicocele." This urologist questioned whether the previous one had taken an ultrasound. Bill explained that an ultrasound had never been mentioned as a diagnostic option. This urologist then asked the couple if it would be all right if he got Lisa in to see one of the reproductive endocrinologists at the medical center while they were there. Lisa recalled, "I'd seen so many doctors, I thought, *What does it matter?* I was frustrated that the doctor I was working with wanted to start over from scratch, and was unsure enough to want to see someone else. I told him I would do it, which is really kind of amazing, because it would have taken me months just to get in to see someone if I had started the procedure. The way it was, I got in the next day."

While Bill was in surgery, Lisa went to her appointment with the reproductive endocrinologist, Doctor K. She and the doctor discussed the options, all the way up to in vitro fertilization (IVF). Lisa had discussed IVF with her first reproductive endocrinologist, but at that time she had thought that if the problem reached that extreme, she would never consider the procedure. She said, "I couldn't imagine spending that kind of money on something with those odds of success. Once we got to that point, I thought, that would be it."

Prior to Bill's surgery, his doctor had told him and Lisa that he wanted to remove the spleen, because it would be difficult to diagnose any problem conclusively without removal. This was done, and the doctor came in to discuss the results with Lisa and Bill after the surgery. He told them Bill had a malignancy on his spleen, and that the spleen was being biopsied to determine what type of malignancy they were dealing with. It was later determined that it was a non-Hodgkins, B-cell Lymphoma, and was quite advanced. The doctors had also removed Bill's appendix because they had found an abnormal node on it. They also biopsied several areas in the abdomen and found abnormal cells in his blood, liver, and bone marrow.

The news crashed in on the couple like a tidal wave. They had been told by the oncologist Bill had seen that the spleen was not cancerous. Their faith in the medical community had been slowly disintegrating, and this experience was truly the last straw. If it had not been for their infertility and Bill's love of flying, the cancer would have gone undiagnosed, and the result could have been Bill's death.

The doctor at the medical center told him he was lucky, because there is a good chance of recovery from lymphomas if they are caught early. But the doctor also said that the type of lymphoma Bill had was abnormal—one so rare that there were not valid studies on recovery rates. Lisa remembered, "I didn't think the odds were very good. I went to the clinic and tried to get every piece of information, to read and absorb it. Bill didn't want to. In fact, when the doctor came in and told us it was cancer, I cried, but Bill did not react to it. The doctor sent me down to lunch, and when I came back up, Bill had made all these phone calls. He had called his doctor in our town and told him everything was fine, and he had called his employers and told them he would be back flying in a couple months after the incision had healed. I asked him if he told them it was cancer, and he said, 'They don't know that yet.' I reminded him that the doctor had just come in and told him he had cancer. He said, 'No, that's not what he said.' He was denying he had cancer, and did not want any information about it."

Bill remembered, "I really did not process that I had cancer until later that night. It's strange—I heard the news, but I didn't comprehend it."

In the face of this health threat, Bill and Lisa's infertility became a back-burner issue. Their concerns lay with accepting and fighting the cancer, reviewing legal documents, preparing for the possibility of Bill's death, and loving their small son. Lisa said, "In that time I had to try and figure out a way to deal with our situation and keep to myself, because I couldn't talk to him about it. I couldn't talk to anybody else about it, because I didn't want anyone going to him and saying, 'Oh, I hear the odds aren't very good.' That was a real pressure: trying to deal with that and having to think about kids. I was so glad that I had seen that reproductive endocrinologist, because he recommended that we bank sperm before the chemotherapy."

Bill had banked some sperm at the regional medical center. Lisa said, "For him I think he felt it was the end of the line—no more kids. For me, I said, 'Bill, it's my life, too.' I wanted to have more children. I told him I didn't want to live my life waiting for him to die so I could remarry and have more children. That would crush our marriage. I had thought about the possibility of raising our child alone; there are a lot of single parents in the world today. I told Bill that any time that the child would have with him, whether it's a month, a year, or ten years, would be more valuable than a lot of two-parent family relationships with their children."

A year and six months of chemotherapy later, Bill was cancer-free. Bill said, "When I got the news that I was cancer-free, Lisa was insistent that we resume our attempts at having a child. I felt resentment over that. I didn't need that pressure when I was in the midst of cancer. It's not just another child. I felt that if the cancer returned, it would be another child I would be responsible for that I wouldn't be able to bring up. I just wanted her to give me time. It has been about two years since I've been in remission. I'm about ready for another child now, but I wasn't then. But in deference to her—how can you tell someone you love that she can't have a child?"

A month after the prognosis, Lisa called the regional medical center and expressed interest in having IVF. They informed her that she could be put on the schedule in September, seven months away. Lisa thought, "Gosh, a year ago I had been there and had been approved for the IVF. When Bill had gotten out of the hospital we had gone to the class where they showed you how to give yourself injections to prepare the body for IVF. We'd figured we could wait and call them when we were ready to start—I didn't know we would have to be put on a list."

Lisa saw the embryologist from the regional medical center, Doctor M, and he asked if she had heard that the head physician for IVF was leaving to start his own practice. He then told her that July would be the last cycle of IVFs for the medical center until a new doctor could be hired. The couple questioned their reproductive endocrinologist about it, and he told them that they could do a stimulation cycle in July and record it as a trial to see how Lisa would respond to the stimulation in preparation for IVF. He told Lisa, "If you have several eggs, they are not going to just let you go. They will bring you in for retrieval." Lisa was told that because she would need to be monitored very frequently while on an IVF cycle, she had to be seen in her home town, and that the results would be sent to the team of doctors at the regional medical center. The clinic informed her that they worked with a doctor in her town. Which meant, to her frustration, one more doctor, one more new patient visit, and one more outlandish sum for a new patient visit. As it turned out, the new doctor at the satellite clinic was the reproductive endocrinologist, Doctor F, that she had originally decided not to see. The irony of this was difficult for Lisa to live with.

To prepare her body for the IVF procedure, Lisa needed very potent medication. In July, when Lisa picked up her prescriptions, the cost was approximately twelve hundred dollars. The first prescription was for the drug Lupron. Lisa injected Lupron shots twice daily into her thigh, starting on the third day of her cycle, to suppress the ovaries. Ovary suppression was needed so that when the medication stopped, ovulation would occur on time. Lisa took Lupron for ten days. The doctor then did a baseline ultrasound and estradiol. The stimulation cycle began on day one, after the Lupron shots. Her Lupron dosage was then reduced to an injection in the morning, and she began to take one hundred and fifty units of Metrodin in the morning and seventy-five units in the evening. After three days of this, she started taking one hundred and fifty units of Pergonal. (The medications are used to stimulate the ovaries into producing eggs.) On the seventh day of the stimulation cycle she began having blood tests taken to determine the estrogen level in her body, and had a vaginal ultrasound. Usually, stimulation medication is continued until the optimal development of the follicles (the structures within the ovary that contain the egg) has been achieved.

Lisa remembered, "I went to my home town clinic for my first ultrasound. They didn't talk to me. The doctor talked to the nurse, and it went back and forth. I came home and didn't know what they had been talking about.

"There was one abnormal follicle that the doctor wasn't happy with. His nurse called me at three in the afternoon and told me they had another ultrasound scheduled for the next day, and that I should be ready to go for egg retrieval. Bill would have to make out his schedule a month in advance, and it was such a guessing game to predict when I was going to ovulate. He never knew how to fill out a schedule. I called Bill at work and told him that they had advised me to be prepared to go for egg retrieval."

Lisa was dizzy with the thought that in a few days she would be able to see her future baby in a petri dish, waiting to be united with its mother. She was elated about the upcoming procedure; in a few short days she believed she could be expecting a baby. She wanted desperately to share her news with the world, but from her previous experiences, Lisa knew that it was not a good idea. She said, "I was just giddy, and I had this huge smile on my face. Yet at the same time I didn't talk to my mom, Chris, about it; this was because of her reaction when I told her I was going to take Clomid. She said, 'Oh Lisa, I wish you wouldn't do that. I just want you to have one baby—I don't want you to have a whole litter.' That just cut me to the quick. Then she went on to say, 'I just wish you would adopt.' I thought, *She has five kids, and this is not her decision.* I told her, 'I didn't come to you to have you make my decisions. I came to you just to talk and to get some support.' If my mom had a hard time accepting that I took Clomid, there was no way I was going to tell her about IVF."

Being able to get support from family and friends during such an intrusive and expensive procedure as IVF is vital for a couple's well being. But Lisa felt she could tell no one. Bill felt frustrated, because he wanted to talk to his parents about the IVF decision, but he felt he could not because Lisa did not want to talk to hers. She recalled, "It wasn't only my mom; there were other people I couldn't tell. When Bill had his cancer, there was another family member who seemed to enjoy being the bearer of bad news. She was the one who told my grandmother about Bill's illness. I hadn't been able to talk about it at the time, and I needed my privacy until I was ready. When I was ready to tell my grandmother, she already knew. I was concerned that if people knew about the IVF, there would be all those stupid remarks to contend with. Comments like, 'So this is your test tube baby, huh?' I felt that this kind of remark made it sound like I wasn't going to have a real baby. It's not plastic, it's not artificial—it's real."

Lisa went in to her clinic for an ultrasound on Friday morning. (At each ultrasound, the size of the follicles were measured. When the follicles reached a certain size, they were mature, and the eggs could be harvested.) She was full of hope, expecting her doctor to give her information on the next step in the process. All he said, however, was that someone would call between three and five that afternoon to tell her which shots she should take. Lisa went home and anxiously awaited her phone call, wondering if tomorrow would be the day to go to the medical clinic. The thought of actually having the IVF thrilled her.

The phone call came and her doctor told her he was going to cancel the cycle because he was not happy with the follicles. There was one abnormal follicle, and he didn't like the way it looked. The follicles varied greatly in maturation; one was quite advanced while the other was much smaller.

As the doctor delivered his news, Lisa listened in disbelief. She remembered, "It was a Friday afternoon, and no one else was around. I thought, *Can't you at least do the artificial insemination? I have spent all this money on medications and I have nothing, nothing at all to show for it, just because of how the timing worked out.* Working with a satellite clinic was a problem—I never got the whole picture. When I talked to the doctors at the medical clinic, they thought that I was getting all the information from the satellite clinic. I was just stuck in the middle, and I was paying double. I was paying the full price at the regional medical clinic plus paying the doctor here in my hometown, only to get a half or a fourth of the information. That was a real frustration for me. I know it would be next to impossible, but if I ever did it again, I would really consider staying with friends to avoid the satellite situation. It just added to the stress. It's expensive enough as it is, and when you add another doctor on it's ridiculous."

Lisa had wanted to at least have artificial insemination done that cycle. Her doctor, however, not only felt that retrieval of the follicle would be a waste of time, effort, and money for Lisa, but he knew that Lisa and Bill had only a few sperm samples available, and therefore did not suggest an artificially inseminated cycle. Lisa said, "Bill and I had a limited amount of monetary resources, though. We knew we couldn't keep coming back and doing the IVF. We had spent twenty-six hundred dollars on medication to stimulate egg production and we now had nothing to show for it.

"I wanted to do the artificial insemination, and the reason we didn't was a miscommunication. When I talked to my doctor at the regional medical center, he told me they could have easily done it."

What many doctors do not seem to realize is that infertile couples need to cling to any chance, no matter how small, of a pregnancy occurring, particularly once their hopes have been raised. Doctors need to be aware of this fact, and should be sure to inform their patients of the range of options. Then they should let the couple make their own decision. Infertile couples need to have control over their medical destiny, and doctors cannot expect the infertile couple to ask about options other than those the doctor has discussed.

After Lisa got off the phone with the doctor from the satellite clinic, she sat in her house all alone. Alone with the news that the IVF procedure that was to finally produce a baby had been canceled. Alone with the realization that this had been the regional medical center's last IVF cycle for some time. Alone with the overwhelming grief. She felt as if the lifeline she had been clinging to had been cut, leaving her floating on a lifeless sea, all alone.

A week after receiving the news of the IVF cancellation, Lisa called the regional medical center. They confirmed that the IVF program would be discontinued for a few months until a new group of doctors came in, and informed her that she would be on the top of the list once the program resumed. Lisa remembered, "They told me I could go back there once the program was reestablished. But the question was, did I want to? When the previous doctors were there they were having seventy-five percent success rates while other places around the country were having twenty-five or thirty percent success rates. The embryologist, Doctor M, told me he had no idea why the statistics were that high. I think it was because the doctors clicked so well together. I kept thinking that this was a ten-thousand-dollar procedure, and it was going to be performed by doctors who had never worked together before. I wondered if that was our most advantageous choice."

Like Lisa, many infertility patients become very attached to the doctors they work with. The attachment can be very strong when the doctors are viewed as competent and caring people. When the doctor/patient relationship is prematurely severed, it can result in a traumatic grief cycle for the patient.

Lisa and Bill decided to contact the team of doctors that had just left the regional medical center. They informed her that they could see her in October, the start of their new partnership's first IVF cycle. But along with moving to a new facility with this team of doctors, she also needed to move to a new satellite clinic.

At her first visit, the team of doctors decided to elevate the dosage of her medication to produce better follicles for this new cycle. More medication meant an increase in cost: the twelve hundred dollar medication bill was now sixteen hundred dollars. Lisa soon started her trips to the hospital for her ultrasound examinations, and she remembered, "It was exciting to see the follicles get bigger every day. I went to almost every examination by myself, but on one of the visits Bill was home and I begged him to come with me. He brought his newspaper and he sat in a chair and read while they were doing the ultrasound. I said, 'Bill, do you see what's going on?' He would briefly look up from his paper and say, 'Oh, yeah.' And that really hurt. I couldn't make him be excited, but this was so exciting and interesting to me. Even though the ultrasound did not show a baby, it was so interesting to see it. I was thinking how amazing it was, and he was sitting there reading his paper.

"I asked the doctor if I could have a picture of the follicles. I explained that I had ultrasounds of my son in utero, and that I wanted to show my next baby his/her first picture. That way I could tell the baby that this was when he/she was an egg and not even a fertilized embryo yet."

The reproductive endocrinologist Lisa and Bill had been working with called and told them it was time for the IVF procedure. The couple checked into the clinic, and Lisa had blood work done as well as another ultrasound to check the progress of the follicles. After the tests, Lisa and Bill saw the clinic's psychologist. They had to decide if they wanted to use cryopreservation on any extra embryos, and they also needed to make a decision on whether or not they would consider using selective reduction; the psychologist would help them explore their feelings around these choices.

With the IVF procedure, embryos are placed in the uterus. Doctors put in more than one embryo to increase the chance of a pregnancy occurring. Sometimes multiple pregnancies occur, and couples are asked if selective reduction is desired. Selective reduction can be done as early as four weeks after fertilization, and is performed to increase the chance of a viable birth. The embryonic sacs can be detected with an ultrasound, and a needle can be inserted into one or more of them to reduce the number of embryos.

Lisa and Bill were asked how many embryos they wanted transferred.

The clinic was averaging six, and Lisa was informed that when the doctors were at the regional medical center, the highest number of children produced from six transferred embryos was triplets. The doctors went on to tell her that during the current cycle, they did have a woman who had four or five live embryos; she and her husband were in the midst of making the decision of whether to use selective reduction.

The doctors wanted Bill and Lisa to very carefully consider the consequences they might face, and as they discussed selective reduction, Lisa thought back to the painful comment her mother had made to her about not wanting "a litter of grandbabies." Lisa recalled confronting her mother about the statement later, and her mother replying, "I'm sorry for making that remark. But all I hear are these stories about women who have to make these difficult choices, and I don't want you to have to make them." Lisa had then thought to herself, *Well, okay; you can understand if I get pregnant and have one baby. But so what if I have five babies? I'd be thrilled to have five babies. If you don't want to come to my house because it's a zoo, that's your choice to make. But it's my choice to have those babies and my choice not to be hurt by those comments.* In that moment, Lisa had known she would never consider selective reduction, because she is vehemently opposed to abortion, and for Lisa, selective reduction was tantamount to abortion.

Bill remembered, "I wasn't sure if we should do IVF. I'm against abortion as well, and I don't like selective reduction. That still concerns me. I really didn't want to be put in that situation. If if would kill the mother, I don't think there is a choice. I said we would use it if Lisa's life was threatened, but I prayed we would not have to."

Lisa told the doctors she would not have a problem with carrying the babies, however many there turned out to be. If she needed to lie flat on her back for the entire pregnancy to carry the babies to term, Lisa would do it. However, Lisa was surprised when Bill said, "If your health was at risk I would not allow that to happen. If it would be healthier for you to reduce the number of embryos, we would do it. Your health is the number one priority." Lisa was amazed at the love in her husband's voice; at that moment she knew that he was committed to her. Infertility had demanded a large toll from their marriage. No longer did they have the fairy-tale marriage they once had. But Lisa felt their love, their marriage, their commitment to each other had been renewed by his statements.

Lisa struggled with her options. Should she ask the doctors to only put three or four embryos within her? Should they go with six embryos and carry however many lived? Should they go with six embryos and use selective reduction if her health and the babies' health were threatened?

Another question was whether they should they tell anyone. If they did tell others, Lisa wondered, would they be judged?

This was the last effort Lisa and Bill could afford, and Lisa desperately wanted to have the best chance possible to become pregnant. After much soul-searching the couple decided to have six embryos transferred and any extras frozen for use later on. Lisa hoped she could have six transferred and six frozen, because the doctors found eighteen follicles. With an egg in each follicle, Lisa felt she would have a good chance of having at least twelve that would be mature.

The next morning Lisa went in for egg retrieval. In this procedure, the eggs are retrieved using transvaginal ultrasound and transvaginal-guided needle aspiration. The needle is inserted into each follicle and draws out first the fluid, and then the egg. Her doctor told her that there was pain involved, but that she would get some 'Don't give a damn' medicine to get her through the procedure. Lisa said, "After the discussion with the doctor, I expected to be very alert. But as I waited to go into the room where the procedure would be done, the girl ahead of me came out of there and looked like she had come out of major surgery. I wasn't ready for that, and I had only two minutes to prepare myself.

"Once the medicine was administered I wasn't out, but I would say I was real close. Even with the medication, though, it was very painful. I was incredibly nervous as I was lying on this table. It felt like someone was pulling a slingshot back and then releasing it right into my uterus. I don't know if the pain came from retrieving the eggs from my follicles or what, but I remember jerking every time it was done. And I kept wondering if my jerking was causing problems. I had tears running down my face and I kept asking for more medicine, but they refused."

After the procedure the doctors told Lisa and Bill they had retrieved nine eggs, and that they were thrilled about it. Lisa, on the other hand, was bitterly disappointed. Her plan for six transfers and six frozen embryos was not possible. Lisa remembered, "I heard the nurse making a comment to someone else that I was actually disappointed about retrieving nine eggs. But I knew they wouldn't all be fertilized, so I wanted more. Afterwards I was taken to another room to recover. The nurse kept telling me to sleep and I kept telling her I was fine. I suppose it was the giddy excitement of it all."

Lisa and Bill went back to their hotel that evening having been informed that in about thirty hours they would be called and told when the transfer would take place. For Lisa, having the retrieval over with and knowing there were eggs available left her feeling that this time was it. This was God's will; her baby—maybe even her twins—were about to be returned to her body.

The wait turned out to be too difficult for a woman who had waited seven years to become pregnant. Lisa ended up calling the clinic asking when she should come in for the transfer. The nurse Lisa talked to was unsure but said she would check, and that if Lisa did not hear any news, she was to come in at eight the next morning. Lisa and Bill waited around the hotel that afternoon for a call, and when they did not receive one, they decided to spend the evening relaxing and rejoicing with close friends.

Lisa remembered being very sore from the retrieval, but the aches paled in comparison to the growing excitement she felt. Lisa and Bill shared the news with their friends and began their evening on a relaxed, positive note. They left the phone number of their friends' home with the clinic, but did not expect it to be used. Later that evening, however, the phone rang and the caller asked for Lisa. It was the head physician. He said, "Lisa, I'm sorry to tell you I don't have very good news." Lisa sucked in her breath and thought, *My husband and I aren't even alone. I'm standing here in my friends' kitchen, everyone is so excited, and then all of a sudden they'll see my face and will know.* The doctor continued, "We put the sperm in with the eggs, and the sperm had a motility of ten percent. The motility was low, but nothing we were concerned about, considering it was frozen sperm. We put them in there, but nothing appears to be happening. We will put another sperm sample in to see if that does anything, but right now we only have one embryo, and it doesn't look that good. It is not a strong, healthy embryo and I don't think it will survive the transfer. We will see what happens in the morning." Trembling, Lisa hung up the phone and gave a short explanation to the group.

Lisa and Bill left for their hotel and spent the night crying, desperately hoping against hope that the embryo would survive and that other eggs would be fertilized. Lisa began reading her Bible study lessons, and as she read them she felt that all of the stories pertained to her. She remembered thinking, *The lessons are all about what I am going through right now. It is going to be all right.* She thought, *Can you imagine the story I'm going to tell? I'll say I had only one embryo, one that was not healthy, but that was all we needed. Just one. This is going to be such a witness to other people, to share my story with them.* Lisa recalled, "I felt so right about it, and I guess that's what I was supposed to do. I don't yet know why it was right, but it was right."

The next morning the doctor called and informed the couple that here was nothing to transfer. The original plan was for the transfer to be done, and then Lisa would rest at the hotel while Bill would go and get a check-up at the regional medical center. Bill had planned to go by himself and return for his wife the next morning, but with the news that there would be no transfer, this plan was no longer necessary. Lisa felt that the cancellation of the transfer was an omen of things to come. She said, "I thought it was a sign. The reason it didn't work was because we were going to the medical center and they were going to tell us Bill's cancer was back."

But the news was good; Bill remained cancer-free. The couple returned home, and as the shock of the failed IVF attempt lessened, Bill and Lisa discussed their options. Prior to the decision to use IVF, Lisa had thought the cost too high and the procedures too extreme. Lisa had felt she could come to terms with the thought of not being pregnant again if she could adopt. Bill, on the other hand, had said it was important to at least try to conceive their baby. It was worth the cost and the effort to him. After the IVF, however, the couple's opinions reversed. Bill was ready to try adoption and Lisa wanted desperately to continue their quest for a pregnancy.

The couple went back to the clinic to discuss the failure of the IVF attempt and future options. The doctor told Lisa, "If I could pick an ideal candidate for IVF, you are it. You're young, you have a child already, you responded well to the stimulation; everything is in your favor. The only thing is, I wouldn't do it again with Bill's sperm. If we did, I really believe the results would be the same. But if you were able to consider donor sperm, that would be a very realistic option for you." (It was later mentioned that the use of donor sperm might mean that artificial insemination could be effective in achieving a pregnancy.) For Bill, however, donor sperm was not a consideration at that time. Bill was very uncomfortable about not knowing who the donors were, or their motivations for donating sperm. Another factor in Bill's rejection of donor sperm was that he felt there was too high of a chance of Lisa contracting diseases from the specimen.

The doctor went on to explain the other option available to them—a procedure called micromanipulation. In this procedure, they would take Lisa's egg and drill a small hole in the outer shell so as to make fertilization more likely with Bill's slow-moving sperm. He told Lisa and Bill the clinic would be doing this procedure relatively soon, that there would be only about a five percent chance of a pregnancy, and that the cost would be approximately twenty thousand dollars per attempt. They left the clinic having told the doctor they were unsure of what actions they would take.

On the way home, Lisa's shock began to wear off. As she played back the events in her mind, she felt that while she had been prepared for the IVF, she had not been prepared for the possibility and consequences of not completing the IVF cycle. Also, Lisa said, "I was not prepared at all for the impact of infertility on our sexuality. I blame the IVF procedure, but I don't know for sure that it was the cause. Maybe it was the deadlines we had set up for ourselves. When we got home we couldn't have intercourse for awhile because my ovaries were enlarged from the stimulation. When it was okay for us to resume intercourse, I just couldn't. I could step outside myself and let my husband have my body, but I could not make love to him. I was afraid I was always going to hate sex for the rest of my life, and I mourned for that. It would be the biggest slap in the face I could get, because every time that I have sex it is not making love, it is just sex.

"God gave us the ability to make love and create life. I knew that this body couldn't make babies, and yet I felt I had to go through the motions. I felt so degraded and bad, and yet here is my husband who needs to feel reassured that a baby isn't everything to me, and who needs me to love him. I told myself I would never say no to him, but every time he would just start to touch me the tears would soak my pillow. Finally Bill said, 'If you need a little time, that's okay. I won't wait forever, but I will wait.'

I think that was one of the greatest gifts of love he could ever give me; I think it would have been very damaging to me if I would have continued to have sex in that way.

"Two or three weeks later I had the ability to come to him once again with a true desire, and for that I am grateful. But in no way was I prepared for this to be a part of our infertility. The ironic joke at our house is that sex creates babies. We know that's a joke, because when you are infertile and trying to have a baby you never conceive by sex."

Lisa remembered that as part of the IVF procedure they were seen by a psychologist prior to the egg retrieval. She said, "We talked about options and our comfort level with the procedure. We had no problems that we needed to talk to her about at that time; we were so excited about our future. That was not when I needed a psychologist. I needed to talk to her when the IVF didn't work. I needed her when I began resenting my body and withdrawing from my husband. That option was not available to us as part of the treatment." Lisa feels that ongoing counseling would be very beneficial to infertile couples as part of their medical treatment, and that the fee should be included in the medical costs. Lisa said, "There are always emotional issues that you need to talk about. No one tells you what to expect, and although our doctors gave us the answers when we asked them, there were times when I couldn't ask the questions because I was emotionally devastated. So the questions remained unanswered."

Lisa and Bill realized that the strain of infertility and the failed IVF cycle had affected their marital relationship deeply. They felt it was time to find someone who could help them deal with their anger, depression, and loss, and they felt that the counselor needed to be a Christian. The couple heard of a Christian marriage seminar that was being held in another state, so they went to it and later talked with the counselor, James, privately. They wanted to talk with him alone because they had learned that he and his wife had dealt with infertility for nine years. Lisa and Bill wanted his help in finding some answers and some resources. Lisa remembered feeling elated that they had found a kindred soul, someone who had experienced the hellish pain of infertility. She was certain he could shed some light upon their situation and offer advice on how they could start healing themselves and their marriage.

Lisa and Bill explained their situation to the counselor. After they finished, James said, "The obvious question is: Why don't you adopt?" Lisa recalled sensing that James felt the issue was so simple, and that he was questioning their need to deal with their infertility. Lisa said, "As he asked about why we hadn't adopted, I thought, *It's not that simple. Babies aren't exactly falling out of trees these days.* However, the counselor went on to explain that he and his wife had four lovely children, all adopted. He said that adoption was the answer, and that the process of adopting was simple. He explained that just days before a young woman had come to his office and said that she was expecting a baby in two months. She wanted to give the baby up for adoption. As Lisa heard the news she became excited, thinking he was mentioning this as an opportunity for them. Lisa started asking about what they would need to do to pursue an adoption with this woman, but the counselor said, "Oh, well, that baby is coming too soon—you wouldn't have time." Later he confessed that he and his wife were interested in adopting the baby themselves. Instead of leaving with a feeling of being rejuvenated, Lisa left feeling cheated.

As this is being written, Lisa and Bill are actively looking for a resolution to their infertility. Part of achieving that resolution means being honest and acknowledging each other's feelings. At this point, Lisa desperately wants to become pregnant. She said, "Our problem now is the male factor. More than anything I wish donor sperm could be an option for us, but it isn't an option for Bill. There is a part of me that resents his feelings about donor sperm. I resent that he will not at this point even consider it, but I also understand and respect his right to his feelings. I think Bill resents that I want donor sperm to be an option.

"I have one child and I desperately want this other child. There are not a lot of people who could come up with the money to try micromanipulation—that is our other option besides adoption. But we could. It would mean sacrificing; sacrificing our lifestyle and cutting out travel and new vehicles. Still, we could handle it. But now, all of a sudden, Bill tells me I'm asking for too much. I have one child, and he asks me why I'm not happy with that. I respond by reminding him of the conversation we had prior to our marriage. I told him I wanted at least two children. Having only one was never one of my choices. Why do I have to feel guilty? It's important enough to me to fit the expense of the procedure into our budget, but it's not to him. We are not on even ground here."

Bill said, "I get stuck in a position I don't like. On one hand I'm the one who is supposed to make the decisions and I'm the one who needs to give her a child. I can't. I can spend money that may allow us to have a child, but what concerns me is where is the limit, how far do we go? I still desire another child, but I feel she has been pushing, pushing, pushing me. I resent that pressure because I can't get away from it. I don't like being pushed, but she's looking at her biological clock—and I realize that. When you start spending significant amounts of money on failed treatments—it's hard not to think about whether we are jeopardizing our retirement account or tuition for my son's college. I feel she doesn't want to face the money issue. Her idea is that things will work out—it's almost like she's avoiding it."

In the months that followed the failed cycle of IVF, a number of things took place. Lisa went to Doctor F, the reproductive endocrinologist, complaining of incredible back pain. He performed a laparoscopy and found that more endometriosis had formed, and that it was attached to the nerve endings in her lower back. Most of the endometriosis was removed by laser surgery, and she began taking six months of Lupron shots to help rid her body of what is left. After her last month on Lupron, Bill and Lisa will try to achieve a pregnancy using a super ovulation cycle. She will take medicine to increase egg production, and the few sperm samples that are left from before Bill's cancer treatment will be used to try and artificially inseminate her. Lisa said, "I know our chances are slim, but then I think that God only needs one chance, and it doesn't matter what the odds are. If He wants it to happen, it will."

The couple has also begun pursuing adoption through a private agency. It took Bill awhile before he decided this could be an acceptable option for him. The couple has their application in and will be sending out their portfolio to prospective mothers who are planning to give their child up for adoption. Lisa said, "Adoption is something I have really pushed for, and right now I'm in a lull stage of infertility. I want to adopt, yet I hold out this hope that the artificial insemination will work or that Bill will change his mind about donor sperm. I definitely want a baby. As we work through the adoption process, we have found out that the baby we will get most likely will be at least two months old. It may seem petty, but I want that baby when it is one day old. I don't want someone to have my baby for two months. I know I'll have that baby for the rest of my life, but it's the way I feel. A baby through adoption would be wonderful, but I still hold on to the hope of a pregnancy. I want to be able to give birth again and to nurse my baby. I want those things."

As her words indicate, Lisa is hoping against hope that the artificial insemination will work. She said, "I know I should be careful not to get my hopes too high, yet I know I have to have faith. I feel like I am the persistent woman in Luke:18. The story is about how this woman keeps coming to the judge and asks him to give her what she desires. Finally the judge tells her that he will grant her desires, not because she is right, but because she is persistent. I know you can move a mountain if you believe. I want to believe I will have a baby. I want to have faith. But truthfully, I don't know what I should believe. I don't know what will be in Bill's and my future. I do know that I will ask God to help us get through to the day when both Bill and I can be completely happy again. That is the day I am looking forward to."

One reason Lisa and Bill decided to tell their story was because by doing so, they hope others can find that the feelings they may be experiencing are not abnormal. They want others to know that their marriage will be affected and that men and women handle their grief in very different ways.

Bill suggested, "I think people need to understand that we, as individuals, are responsible for our own health care. For instance, I was told I had a varicocele, and I didn't. If any man is told that he has a varicocele, he should demand that an ultrasound be performed—it may save him an unnecessary surgery. Also, I highly recommend getting a second opinion—I think it should be a matter of course. I wouldn't be here if I hadn't obtained one."

Lisa said, "I want people to know that there are definite traps of infertility to try and avoid. One of those traps is lack of control. The only thing you know for certain is your desire for a baby, and everywhere people are telling you what to do to get that baby, how to feel, and what emotions are appropriate. In the meantime, your marriage is taking an incredible beating. Your partner, the one you love so deeply, may not be on the same wavelength as you. You want to find answers to your problems, but at the same time you don't want the answers because you begin feeling guilty for everything. Guilty for being infertile, guilty for not wanting to accept child-free living or adoption, guilty for being sad, guilty for hoping for a pregnancy, guilty for feeling anything at all. The result is that guilt piles on top of itself and the infertility begins to smother you. That's when couples need to know that this reaction is completely normal. They need to know how important it is to try and accept feelings and not feel guilty about them. Acceptance is a large part of gaining control over infertility."

5

ANGEL'S STORY

Surgical Sterility and Adoption

Sitting in a car overlooking a picturesque lake, Angel told her story. At forty-three she is pretty and vivacious, yet still haunted by the spectre of her infertility.

Angel was left sterile by two surgeries before the age of twenty. Years later, talking about her experience is still very difficult for her. She began by saying, "Most people don't know all of what I'm going to tell you. They think that because I have a child that part of my life is long since over and I have healed completely. It is over, but I still have a lot of feelings buried, and I guess I always will."

Angel has always loved children. She remembers sitting on her father's lap, telling him that when she grew up that there was going to be a mommy and a daddy and a baby living in a house with a white picket fence, and that the mommy was going to be her. She remembered her father stroking her hair and saying, "That may be." The idea of having a child and loving it with the same intensity that she was loved by her parents was a long-term goal for Angel. She never believed that she would be unable to give birth to her baby.

A month after Angel had turned seventeen, she was asked to accompany two friends to a livestock auction and watch their three children while the parents, Darla and John, were busy. Angel remembered the ride home: "I was in a really good mood, and I was talking to John in the car. I had just told him about the new wallet I had, that it was a gift from my brother.

"John and Darla sat in the front seat of the car, with their baby between them. The baby was in a car seat—car seats back then served the purpose of keeping a baby still, but not safely restrained. I sat in the back seat behind John, and the two boys sat to my right.

"I noticed that John was driving pretty fast, and I commented on it to him. The last thing he said to me before the accident was, 'At least I'll get you home alive.' I looked out the left window and saw a car coming straight at us. I screamed that the driver had run the stop sign, and a second later the car slammed into my door. Our car rolled three times, and Darla, who was pregnant at the time, and the baby that had been in the car seat were thrown clear of the car. We skidded about one hundred and fifty feet and rolled two more times before the car stopped, upside-down, in a ditch. In the initial impact, John had been thrown back onto me, and I had put my arm around the closest boy's neck and head. I blacked out at some point, and when I came to I saw the car blinkers going. I crawled out of the car and heard the baby crying. As I stepped over to see if he was okay, I collapsed and blacked out again. When I came to the next time there were a lot of cars that had stopped."

One of the cars drove the family and Angel to the hospital. Remarkably, there seemed to be no major injuries; all were examined and released that day. Angel remembered that what had worried her the most had been losing her wallet. The next day her brother Barry took her to the site to search for it. Angel said, "That we all lived was amazing, especially when you consider that John had two cans of gas in the trunk that weren't sealed. I was naive, though, and my main concern was losing my wallet. After Barry told me he couldn't find it, I bawled.

"When we were driving home, I became petrified with fear. Barry saw my reaction and started speeding down a gravel road—he told me that I needed to get over my fear, and this would help me do it. Looking back on it, I think it did. Three weeks later, a similar accident to ours occurred in the same place, and two people died."

Angel had in fact suffered a lot of damage from the accident, but it went unnoticed at first. Up until the accident, Angel's periods had been sporadic, but afterwards they became increasingly heavy, and she began to pass large clots of blood. Angel remembered, "I started my period, and after ten days of flowing heavily, I started marking my calendar. I was very frightened that something was really wrong with me—I would flow through two maxi pads within a short amount of time. I was afraid to tell my folks, so I started using my lunch money to buy sanitary protection for myself. After each class was over I would ask my girlfriend to check my clothes to see if I was bleeding through my outfit. A number of times I found that I was.

"After forty days of flowing, my mom came to my room and saw that my calendar was marked with x's. When she questioned me about their significance, I said, 'I don't know.' Her first thought was that I was pregnant. After I told her what was happening, she took me to a doctor."

After hearing about the symptoms Angel was having, the doctor prescribed birth control pills to regulate her period and reduce the flow. At the time, no mention was made of the accident because Angel did not suspect a connection between the two events. Angel said, "Everything was okay until the kids at school found out. When it got around that I was on birth control pills they pointed fingers at me and accused me of sleeping around. Those days were filled with humiliating statements, and I really had a hard time dealing with their ignorance."

The prescription seemed to help, but by May of the next year, Angel starting having incredible pelvic pain. She remembered, "A few days before graduation we were practicing a song for the ceremony. I felt so bad that day, and finally some of my friends took me up to the hospital. When Mom and Dad got there I was vomiting green bile, sweating with a fever, and was as white as a ghost. Because of my condition, doctors were called out of surgery to examine me. I was scared enough as it was, and when I saw these doctors that were covered in blood from head to toe, I just started freaking out.

"The doctors didn't know what was wrong with me. They took blood tests and all that. They finally decided to do exploratory surgery to try to determine why I was so sick. They found that one of my ovaries had wrapped around my appendix three times. They said that my internal organs were very jumbled, and attributed it to the accident the previous summer. They removed my appendix—not because it was bad, but because it was in that general neighborhood.

"The doctor who did the surgery commented that the ovary is usually the size of an almond. The one that had wrapped around my appendix was closer to the size of a baseball, and was transparent. And of course there were cysts and blood clots on it. They removed the ovary and the fallopian tube, and they also removed a few cysts that were on the other ovary. This whole time was very scary for me, and I was in so much pain that I never questioned what the doctors were doing to me."

After the surgery, Angel's period became more normal. Her life started to look very promising; by age nineteen, Angel had gone to beauty school and had a job as a hair stylist. She was involved in a relationship with a man named Darryl. The two were inseparable, and were starting to discuss marriage. Then one winter evening, as Angel was leaving work, she fell on ice-covered steps and landed on her bottom. Angel remembered, "I landed very hard and it knocked the wind out of me, but as I sat there I started feeling better. I had mild pain Friday evening and Saturday morning, but was not concerned. The pain started to increase Saturday afternoon, though, and by Monday the pain was so excruciating that I went to the emergency room. They did not know what was causing the pain, and I was losing a tremendous amount of blood."

A doctor took Angel into surgery, where he broke her pelvic bone in order to insert his hand and feel the remaining ovary, and to look at the reproductive organs. He told her afterwards that everything appeared normal, and Angel was kept in the hospital for observation. The next day, however, Angel was in more pain than the day before. She was experiencing incredible stomach pains and had red streaks across her abdomen— a sign that she had blood poisoning. Angel recalled, "At that point I was losing blood very fast; in fact, I was bleeding internally. They needed to give me three pints of blood before they could even think of taking me into surgery.

"Rather than sending me away to a specialist, my parents opted to have me stay there. My boyfriend wanted me to be seen by a specialist, but my parents had faith in the doctor that I was seeing. I was so sick that I really did not know what was going on. I remember the doctor coming in and saying to me that there might be a chance I could never have children. I looked at him and said, 'No, no. That can't be.'

"I was kept so drugged out that I had no control over anything. When I'd come to they would shoot me up some more. I do remember going back into surgery, though. A friend of mine had a boss who donated a pint of blood, my brother donated a pint, and I got a pint that was donated by an Amish group. I really had some good feelings about the surgery, that it was going to be a-okay. Still, I remember telling the nurse, 'I'm so scared.' She looked at me and said, 'It's okay, mother's here.' Those were her last words to me before they put me under. I was in surgery for quite some time.

"When I woke up I was really sore. They had done a really big number on me—twenty-some stitches in my stomach. The doctor came in and sat down; he also told me the surgery went well. Then he said, 'We had to go ahead and take your other ovary. We also took a tube, and we tied the other one. You still have your uterus, but the only way you could get pregnant now would be by a freak accident. We wanted to leave you with some organs so you could retain your femininity.'

"I lay there hearing his words and looking right in his eyes, and I could hardly move. Then—I don't know where it came from—I sat straight up in bed and I started to pound on him. I said, 'You dirty rotten son-of-a-bitch! How could you do this to me?' He forced me back down on the bed, and I remember him telling the nurse to do something with the IVs. In a matter of seconds I was unconscious. For the next five or six days I was sedated, drifting in and out of consciousness.

"When I went into the hospital I had weighed approximately one hundred and sixty pounds, and they kept me there about twelve days. In that time I lost about thirty-five pounds."

During the days before her dismissal from the hospital, her boyfriend, Darryl, was with her constantly. He spent the days bringing her presents, holding her hand, and talking about their future. On the day Angel was to be discharged, her brother Barry and a friend of his came to take her home. As they were loading the car with flowers and gifts, Angel's doctor came in. She remembered, "I was still pretty upset about what had happened. At that time there was no counseling or anything. You just had to do what you had to do, get out of the hospital and live with it. That was it.

"No one seemed to understand the impact of what had happened to me. My life had been monumentally altered, and my doctor was saying, 'If you can get out of bed and walk to the door, I'll let you go home.' I was so determined to get out of that damn hospital that although I was barely able to move, I put on my housecoat and walked to the door. I thought, 'God, just get me back to that bed and I'll be all right.' When I reached the bed I said, 'I did it.' I was so out of breath I could barely speak. All my doctor said was, 'Fine. Just sign yourself out when you leave.' There was no compassion or remorse from the doctor, or any of the medical personnel."

When Barry came back from loading the car he told Angel he and his friend would return for her in half an hour, giving her time to get dressed. When he returned, however, Barry and his friend found Angel still sitting in the exact spot where he had left her. Angel begged Barry to help her get dressed so she could leave this unfeeling place that had robbed her of her fertility. Unfortunately, no one had bothered to bring Angel any clothes other than the ones she wore when she entered the hospital. Since then she had lost thirty-five pounds, and her clothes no longer fit. Angel wore those clothes home anyway, holding the waist of the pants to keep them from falling to her ankles.

When Angel got out of the hospital, it was more than her clothes that no longer fit. Her old life also did not fit any longer. She was nineteen, afraid, angry, and sterile. And just as no one had brought her new clothes that fit, no one tried to help her adjust to the changes in her life. No one was there to help her with the devastation; through the entire hospital stay and recovery period, nobody mentioned what had happened to her. Visitors came to see her, but no one inquired about her emotions—they came and left treating her as if she had fallen and broken a bone. No one acknowledged that this was a loss deeper than anything Angel had ever known. Cards were sent that told her to get well. Angel remembered thinking, *How in the world can I get well now?*

Angel went home to recover, and fell into a very dark depression. Angel recalled, "I felt very incomplete. I felt that I had been stripped of all my femininity. Because of my love for kids—I have always, always loved kids—I wondered if God was punishing me. I thought back to the time that I first learned where babies came from. I remember thinking, *I don't ever want kids. It's going to hurt too much to deliver them.* I thought back to that and wondered, *Did God hold me to that? I was just a kid—I didn't mean it.* So many thoughts were running through my head and I didn't know how to feel better. After all, I was never going to have a baby born to me. In one split second, that right had been surgically removed."

Angel's feelings of inadequacy as a woman were soon to be reinforced by Darryl. Angel remembered, "After I got out of the hospital I didn't see

Darryl. I really needed him. Then, two nights after I moved back home, I saw his car parked in front a girlfriend's house. I called the next day and he said, 'We're through, and this is the end of it.' He broke up with me right over the phone. Later I found out that he had broken off our engagement because he wanted children—children I could no longer give him. He was an only child, and he wanted a son to carry on his family name.

"I was horrified when he broke up on the phone with me. After all, he had slept in the waiting room and been so supportive of me in every way. But when I needed him the most, he wasn't there. I had already felt incomplete, so when he broke up with me it seemed like one more event that proved I was. I kept thinking, *Am I ever going to feel good again, am I ever going to be married, am I ever going to be a mother?*"

Particularly painful to Angel was the reaction of her family. Angel reflected, "Infertility and sterility at nineteen is so hard. The body has matured, but the mind and emotions haven't. You don't have the coping skills to deal with a life-long loss.

"My brother was a teacher, educated and bright, but he could not help emotionally. He did not help me survive because he didn't know how. We were a very close family and had an understanding of love. But it took this experience to see that even though we loved each other, we were not connected to each other's feelings. Some of the things that my family said or did not say ended up leaving scars. I remember my mom told me, 'If you were meant to have children you would have had them a long time ago.'" This hurt Angel in a way that little else had, for her mother was insinuating that Angel had been promiscuous. This left her feeling emotionally vulnerable. Angel said, "I was not free with my love like other people thought I was. I never had been. I was nineteen when I lost my virginity, and I lost it to a man that I really had deep feelings for.

"Nobody in my family knew how to deal with the fact of my sterility, so they didn't. Then after I was home for awhile there was a phase where everybody felt so sorry for me. People would come up to me and say, 'Oh, I hear you can't have kids.' It was as if they suddenly felt pity for me. But in the midst of their pity they also wanted to hear about the details."

Angel claimed she really had no idea what the details of her surgery were. She has refused to get her medical records from the hospital. Other doctors have asked to see them, and she has told them she will get them as soon as she is ready. But Angel doubted that she will ever be ready. She said, "I don't want them. I don't want to even see them. I honestly don't know why I don't want to see them; I think maybe it is a phase of my life that I want to forget. I honestly don't know."

Sandy, Angel's mother, believes that the doctor doing the examination inadvertently burst the ovary, and that was the cause of Angel's sterility. Angel said, "I don't know if that was the reason why things turned out the way they did. But I know that to dwell on the tragedy of my sterility would mean I would be forever destined to cry. I feel there is always a reason for something happening. Whether I could have been treated someplace else and still given birth, I don't know. Sometimes I think if that had been the case, maybe the baby might have been stillborn or handicapped, or something might have happened that I couldn't have dealt with. Childbirth possibly could have taken my life. I always feel there is a reason for things that happen."

The emotional impact of sterility left Angel feeling isolated and lost. At times she felt that the grief would eat her alive if she let it. It was at one such point when she began to shut down, to remove herself from the emotional pain of her ordeal. She remembered, "I had looked for someone to help me accept what happened. I had quite a bit of grief, and after finding no help, I just bottled it up inside. My grieving was solitary because I had no one to grieve with me—no one was there to help or explain.

"At that time we were ignorant about the benefits of therapy. You only went to a counselor if you were 'nuts.' I lived through my experience by crying, and by going to places of great beauty; I tried to soak that beauty into my soul. Lots of times I would drive to a lake and imagine that the water was the product of all the tears I had shed. I often thought that I could cry a lake as big as the one I was staring at. I did a lot of soul searching through my writing. I wrote a lot of poems, but I have never, and will never, show them to anyone. They are records of my grief. They will be read by me alone when I need to get in touch with who I was at that point."

In her early twenties, Angel met and married George. Angel had told George of her sterility, and George was very supportive of her. Angel remembered, "George made me feel like I was whole just the way I was. I felt he accepted me.

"Something that was very painful for me happened during our marriage. I wanted a child, and I knew George did too. After a great deal of soul-searching, I called my sister and asked if she would have a baby for me. She told me no, and it almost seemed like she thought I was joking. I wasn't—I was dead serious. Then she gave me her reasons why she couldn't give me a baby. On some level I understood, but on another level I was very hurt.

"After that, George and I talked about adoption—we even picked out names for the children we dreamed of. But our marriage dissolved before we could start the process. Not a lot of people know the reason the marriage ended. It basically was over when I got a call from a woman who told me that she could and was going to give my husband the children that I couldn't." This experience was another slap in the face to Angel. Although there were many things Angel felt she had control over in her life, giving birth to a child was out of her control, and she again grieved for that loss.

Within just a few years, Angel had experienced sterility and a failed marriage. The period after her marriage broke up was one of the most unbearable times she had ever lived through. Angel said she finally overcame the grief by having an epiphany. She said, "I have a secret. The best person to confide in is yourself. I learned that a long time ago; when no one else will listen, listen to yourself. There is no one that knows you better.

"I use this a lot even today. If I have a problem, rather than laying it on someone else's shoulders, I will look in the mirror and I'll get control of my life. I have become my own best friend.

"In order to get through bad experiences you have to realize you are on your own. You have to realize that no one can really be there for you. A lover, spouse, best friend, sister, or parent might be present, but they can't do for you what you need to do for yourself. My faith in God is very, very strong. He talks through me, to me. He is there if you want Him. God can do so much, but you need to take the first steps."

With her new realization, Angel began to feel better about herself and her life. A few years later, she married Ronny. Ronny was very supportive of Angel, and during the first year of their marriage, their pastor informed them that a Lutheran social agency was opening up their waiting list for infant adoptions. The pastor gave them the information on how to begin the process. Angel remembered, "You had to call in to be one of the one hundred couples eligible to get on the waiting list. For three hours straight we called on different phones. (This was before the advent of automatic dialing.) We finally got through; we were the ninety-seventh caller. We had started calling at seven in the morning and we got through at ten. I had to go to work at eight, so Ronny kept calling. When he called me at work and told me that he had gotten through, I was flying high.

"We had to wait until the agency contacted us before we started their required parenting meetings. They put us in groups of six couples. We stayed together, ate together, did everything together as a group for three days straight."

After the weekend training session, a social worker did a personal interview. In the interview the case worker asked what characteristics the couple wanted in an adopted child. The case worker told the couple that some people have a sex preference, want children whose birth parents had particular interests or hobbies, or would like a specific ethnic background. Angel remembered thinking that being 'so picky' was the silliest thing she ever heard of. She said, "I felt that if the child was breathing and wanted to be loved, that was enough. Some of the people we knew had very definite specifications, even up to asking for a child who came from parents that loved music. All I put on our sheet was that we would like a girl who was a newborn or younger. The 'or younger' was an attempt at humor; I didn't realize at the time that agencies such as that one don't have a lot of humor."

After the case worker had completed the interview and left, Angela and Ronny were very diligent in keeping in touch with her. Five weeks after the retreat they learned that the first couple had gotten their baby. Angel remembered, "We were so happy for them, yet we were so jealous because ours wasn't with us yet. Most of the people in our group wanted boys, and boys were more readily available.

"As I waited for the call I wondered how I would react when I got it. Part of me thought I would handle the announcement serenely, while the other part thought I would go bonkers and be very excited. In the months we waited for the call we had moved, and between the two addresses we had three different nurseries set up for our baby.

"It was almost nine months to the day of the retreat that we got the call from the social worker. I got it at two-thirty in the afternoon. She said, 'I have a daughter for you.' And I said, 'Well, isn't that nice? How big is she?' The social worker told me, and then I proceeded to question her about all sorts of little tidbits. I asked when we could get our daughter, and she said we couldn't pick her up the next day because her schedule was full. I immediately said, 'What if we come really early, can we get her then?' She agreed, and I told her we'd see her early the next day."

As Angel hung up the phone she remembered feeling like she was on a nice little cloud. She remembered, "I hung up the phone and thought, 'Oh good, tomorrow I get my daughter.' And then I thought, 'What the hell do I do now?' I tried to call my husband, but his line was busy. He had had a couple of minor accidents at work in the past few weeks and I thought if I called him with the news he might get so excited that he might not be able to keep his mind on work. I knew he would be home in a half hour anyway, and I could tell him then. In the meantime, I thought, *I've got to call somebody. Who do I tell?* I considered calling my mom, but then I thought that wouldn't be fair because Ronny's mom wouldn't know about it. After thinking a little longer, I decided I would call my sister in California and tell her about it. I called and said, 'Guess what? I'm going to be a mother tomorrow.' She got very excited and started asking questions like what color eyes my daughter had. In my excitement, I answered 'two.' She went on to ask me more questions, and I answered them all. I said goodbye, hung up the phone, and then it rang immediately. It was my social worker, and she asked me if I had calmed down yet. I told her I had. She told me the things I would need to get for the baby. I wrote them down and then told her I had gone loco being there all by myself with the news. I remember her laughing, and I felt like I was the most incredibly lucky woman in the world."

Forty-five minutes later, Ronny walked through the door. Angel asked him if he would like to go to Sioux City, fifty miles from their town, the next day. Angel remembered, "He gave me a funny look and asked me why I wanted to go. I told him I thought it might be fun to pick up our new daughter. He looked at me and said, 'This is not a joking matter.' I said, 'I'm not joking.' And he hugged me like I had never been hugged before. We went and told his boss and asked for some time off. His boss said, 'I'll give you a half hour off to go and get the baby and come back.' Then he laughed and took us out to dinner to celebrate."

The next morning the couple drove to Sioux City. Angel brought an embroidered quilt she had made and a little bag they had packed for their daughter. They got to the social worker's office on time and waited outside. Angel remembered, "I looked at my husband and he looked at me, and all of a sudden we saw this elderly woman come in. She had this little bundle in her arms. I said to my husband, 'Is that our baby?' And he said, 'I think so.' Soon after that our social worker came out and asked if we would like to meet our daughter. By this time the tears were already falling down our faces. I walked in and Renea was lying there on the desk in little boy's clothes. Renea was very tiny. I said, 'Oh my God, thank you.' I picked her up and she didn't cry; she kind of meowed.

"We had brought all these different clothes for her. We ended up putting a size zero on her, and it turned out to be really big. Then the foster mother came in; she was the elderly woman we had seen earlier. She asked if we had any questions. The foster mother had only had her for a week, because Renea had been in intensive care for five weeks—she had been delivered prematurely. The foster mother told us that Renea was a wonderful baby and really loved her baths. When it came time for her to leave, I hugged her and thanked her for taking care of our baby. It was the most wonderful feeling to finally be a mother."

The social worker asked Angel and Ronny what they were planning to name their daughter, and why they had chosen the name. The couple explained that they found the name in a baby book. In the book, Renea was listed as meaning "the messenger of God." Angel explained that she felt her daughter was her own personal messenger of God. Renea's middle name, Louisa, was after Angel's grandmother. They told the social worker they had not made a final decision on a name until they were on their way down to get her. Then the couple and the social worker had a spiritual time during which the social worker prayed for the couple and for Renea. Angel remembered, "We wrapped Renea up and walked to the door, and all four of us were crying and in a huddle. Ronny told me, 'You have made me the happiest man in the world.' And then we left."

Angel tucked Renea in the crook of her arm that night so the baby could sleep with her. She was so in love with the baby that she couldn't bear putting her in a crib in another room. She said, "What a lot of people don't understand about adoption is that it fulfills the parenting need. I bonded with this child long before we were on a waiting list, long before she even existed. When I took Renea to the doctor for a checkup, the doctor asked me where she was sleeping, and I told him. He told me to put the baby in a crib, because I might roll on her. He didn't know that I never would have—I had steeled myself to be my baby's rock, her security. But I later put her in a cardboard box on the floor by my bed. The doctor later told me not to do that either. But from the time I first saw Renea it was instant motherhood for me."

Since that time, much has happened in Angel's life. When Renea was three, Angel and Ronny tried to adopt another child, but could not get on the waiting list. After that, Angel asked Ronny if he would support her in finding an egg donor. It was her desire to have an egg fertilized by his sperm, and then carry his baby within her body. Ronny told her that he felt he did not want to risk her health on trying such a procedure. When Renea was six, the couple's marriage dissolved.

Angel has since married a man named Rob. The couple has been married for four years, and both Angel and Rob are extremely happy raising their daughter Renea. Angel has broached the topic of adoption and egg donors to Rob, but he has told her that he is not interested in raising any other children. He feels that Renea is his daughter, and raising her has satisfied his need to parent.

Angel feels the experiences she has lived through have made her a stronger mother. She said, "The one constant in my life is Renea, just as I have been the one constant in her life. Never could I have dreamed of being so close and so in tune with a child. When people tell me, 'You should be proud of your daughter,' I reply, 'I am. I have put sixteen years into her life.'

"I have talked to my daughter since the time she was born about being adopted. I told her, 'You grew in another lady's stomach, but you grew in my heart.' She is my one true joy and I love her dearly."

"I have found that life can be very hard, and that life changes you. When I think about becoming sterile, I know I still haven't accepted it. I have locked the pain and the loss away in a very deep place. It might not be the healthiest thing, but that was my only choice twenty-some years ago. I know I will always have that deep desire for children. As a matter of fact, I just read that the Lutheran agency we adopted Renea from has opened their waiting list. My heart took a blow when I read what the requirements were. They said that to be eligible, an individual had to be forty-two or younger. I am forty-three. They say I'm too old.

"It has been a long time since I lost my fertility, but I still feel the pain. I still feel the loss. The anguish is always right below the surface. My daughter has filled my heart with so much joy and wonder, but she cannot take away my feelings of sadness that surround my sterility."

6

MONTE AND ELAINE'S STORY
Surrogacy

Monte and Elaine grew up in an isolated farming community in the mid-west. They have known each other since they were small children. However, it wasn't until they both left their small town to attend a large university in another state that they began dating. There, amid the hustle and bustle of a bright, exciting new world, they found each other.

"We'd been in school together since the second grade," Elaine said, "but we hadn't connected until college. We drove home together for long weekends and holidays, and we talked a lot on the drive home. We became friends and things just developed from there. He was such a happy-go-lucky guy; I couldn't help falling for him."

Since they both loved literature, Monte and Elaine enrolled in the same English Lit class in their senior year. It was midway through the semester when Monte devised a way to ask Elaine to marry him.

Their instructor always came in the room approximately ten minutes before class, adjusted the overhead projector, and put her first transparency on. She would then turn off the projector, go out in the hall, and chat with students until the bell rang before coming in and turning the overhead on once again. One day, Monte waited until the instructor had gone into the hall and replaced the transparency with one of his own. As the bell rang, the instructor greeted the class and turned the overhead on. Elaine remembered, "I was looking down at my notebook when I heard the class roar with laughter. I looked up and saw the transparency. It said, 'Elaine, I love you. Will you marry me?' At that point the instructor said, 'Elaine, just so you know, this isn't my transparency.' Again, the class howled with laughter. 'Why don't you give us your decision, and then we'll get on with class.' I put my hand to my head and said, 'How can I refuse?' Monte stood and bowed, and the class applauded. I was so embarrassed, but it touched me very deeply."

They married after graduation and both found jobs in a city in their home state. Monte took a teaching position in an elementary school, and Elaine went to work for an engineering firm. In lieu of a large wedding, the couple's parents got together and gave them ten thousand dollars to use however they chose. Monte and Elaine were amazed at their parents' generosity and decided to use the gift as a down payment for a house.

After six months of searching, the couple found their dream house, and once the final papers were signed, they began moving boxes over to their new home. The next day, Elaine's boss informed her that he had chosen her to represent their firm at a large sales meeting in Chicago. Elaine remembered, "Ordinarily I would have been very pleased to have been chosen to go, but we were right in the process of moving. I came home from work extremely irritated and told Monte the news. I said that if he wanted me to come home in a cheerful mood, he had better unpack the boxes in the living room so there would be at least one uncluttered place in the house when I got home."

Three days later Elaine was driving home from the airport, hoping that Monte had not goofed off and had actually cleared out the living room. Elaine said, "As I opened the door I found the living room exactly as I had left it, so I yelled for Monte as loudly as I could. When he didn't answer I assumed he was still at work. I was so disgusted as I looked around the room—there wasn't even a place to sit down. At that point, however, I saw that Monte had unpacked the TV and VCR. How typical! Then I saw a videotape sitting on the VCR with a note attached to it. The note said, 'Play me.'"

Elaine put the tape in the VCR and saw her husband and his third grade class appear on the screen. Monte smiled and said, "Guess you've seen I didn't get to the living room. Sorry. Instead, my class and I have cooked up a little surprise for you. Kids, can you tell her what it is?" Monte stepped off camera and his class came into focus, reciting, "First comes love, then comes marriage, then comes baby in a baby carriage." The children dissolved from focus in a pool of embarrassed giggles. Monte came back on screen and said, "How 'bout it, Elaine? Go down to the last bedroom in back and let's talk."

Elaine shut the TV off and ran to the back bedroom. The door was closed and was plastered with children's drawings of babies. When she opened it she found that the room had been set up as a nursery. She remembered, "I opened the door and I couldn't believe it. Everything was there. The walls were covered with Mickey Mouse wallpaper, a bright red carpet was on the floor, a wooden rocking chair with a pink and blue afghan laying over its back sat in the corner, and in the middle of the room was a canopied crib. Monte, however, was nowhere in sight. As I looked around the room a second time, the closet door opened and out popped Monte and my sister Jackie. They were wearing Mickey Mouse hats and big cloth diapers over their slacks. They looked so silly that I started laughing so hard I almost wet my pants."

It took some time for Elaine to calm down enough to seriously consider Monte's proposal. "I'd been thinking along the same lines, but hadn't brought it up. I wanted babies, but I worried that it might be too early—that maybe we hadn't had enough time to ourselves, but Monte said, 'We can't let this nursery go to waste,' and I agreed."

Three months later Elaine learned she was pregnant. She recalled wracking her brain to try to top Monte's creativity in telling him of her pregnancy. Monte remembered, "I got up to get ready for work, and when I got to the kitchen I found that Elaine had set the dining room table. I knew something was up, because Elaine normally doesn't cook. She told me she had fixed me breakfast because it was 'King for a Day' day. I had started getting excited about a homemade breakfast when she put a bowl of cereal in front of me. Disappointed, I put the spoon in the cereal, and it hit something. I put my fingers in the bowl and fished out a tiny glass bottle. I removed the stopper and read the note inside—it said she was pregnant. I was really happy I was going to be a daddy."

The couple was elated with the pregnancy; Monte went to all of Elaine's monthly doctor visits. When Elaine started seeing the doctor every two weeks, her sister Jackie went with her so Monte would not have to miss so much work. Elaine said, "Jackie is one of the strongest and most independent women I have ever met. We have always teased her about really wanting to marry and become a housewife. She jokes right back by saying something like, 'Yeah, right after I slit my throat.' She would sit in the doctor's waiting room with me, and I asked her once if she was sure she never wanted to become a mother. Jackie assured me that she did not have a maternal bone in her body and that there was no way she would ever want the responsibility of raising a child. She did say, however, that she would be a very good aunt. Jackie was with me thirty-six weeks into the pregnancy when the ultrasound technician told me I was carrying a boy. She put her mouth to a part of my stomach that had not been covered with ultrasound gel and told him that she was his aunt Jackie and that he'd better buy her lots of presents if he knew what was good for him."

When the time came, Elaine was accompanied into the labor room by Monte and Jackie. "It was an incredible experience, Jackie recalled. "Elaine was turning seven shades of blue as she pushed the baby out, and Monte looked like he was going to pass out. The experience was so memorable and I'm glad she asked me to share her pregnancy with her." After being in labor ten hours, Elaine gave birth to her son, Derek John.

Monte and Elaine took Derek home, and both were very proud of their new son. Monte said, "It was like a fairy tale. I had a beautiful wife, a good job, and a wonderful baby. I was so proud of Derek that I brought him into class six days after he was born to meet my kids. Every time he passed gas the kids would scream with laughter. With Derek in my arms my life was complete." Six weeks later, Elaine had to return to work, so she found child care for Derek. Elaine's good friend, Beth, said she would watch him during work days.

Less than three months after their son was born, however, Elaine and Monte's plans for their family's future were irrevocably shattered. Monte remembered, "I was in class, and the principal asked me to step out in the hall. He told me Beth had called, and said the paramedics had taken Derek to the hospital. I froze—I didn't know what to think. I thanked him and drove to the hospital right away. When I got there Elaine and Beth were in an embrace. I knew it was bad, because both of them were crying. I ran to Elaine, and when she saw me she said, 'He's gone, Monte.' She fell into my arms, and we both broke down. The doctor came and said that Beth had put the baby down for a nap at nine that morning and when she checked on him at nine-thirty he wasn't breathing. She called 911 and started doing CPR on Derek. The paramedics came, and upon his arrival at the hospital, Derek was pronounced dead. The doctor felt Derek died of sudden infant death syndrome.

"After the doctor talked to us, Elaine and I went in to see Derek. If I hadn't known better I would have thought he was sleeping. He looked so peaceful, so beautiful. A counselor came in and suggested that we each have our picture taken with him, as our last reminder of our son. They took my picture as I kissed my son goodbye for the last time.

"I don't know how we made it through that day."

Even now, Elaine barely remembers the time at the hospital. She said, "Everything seems like such a blur; I don't remember a whole lot. I remember the doctor telling me that Derek could not be revived, and Beth becoming hysterical, saying that Derek's death was her fault. I remember seeing Derek and saying goodbye to him. After that the doctor prescribed some medication to calm me down.

"I awoke that night thinking I had heard Derek cry. I went into the nursery, and as I turned on the light and looked at the empty crib, I fully realized my baby was dead. I screamed and cried for what seemed forever. I have never known such intense sorrow. I remember thinking that if Derek was dead, I wanted to die too."

The days preceding Derek's funeral were filled with the details of making funeral arrangements, family and friends offering their condolences, and a general feeling of disbelief. Jackie remembered, "When I heard about the news, my first thought was for Elaine, not for Derek. I knew that this baby was everything to her. Whenever she talked about him, her face would light up like a Christmas tree. Derek had been Elaine's world, and now that world was gone.

"Watching Monte and Elaine get through the planning for his funeral was so hard. They were like zombies, making decisions but not really processing anything. I remember telling Elaine that I loved her and that I would do anything in the world for her."

After the minister spoke at the funeral, Monte got up to talk about his son. Monte remembered, "I wanted Elaine to talk, but she was just too distraught. I really don't remember my words, but I remember looking at the sea of faces before me. I looked at my son's white casket and I felt an imperceptible change in the church; when I looked back I didn't see faces anymore—I just saw grief. I think when a child dies, it is the cruelest death of all. I think everybody felt it that day. I told our friends how I was going to miss my son. He was the most beautiful person I ever had a chance to meet, and I felt graced by knowing him. At that point someone started sobbing quite loudly, and I lost whatever composure I had left. Still, I was glad I went up there, because it helped my healing to begin. It was a way to say goodbye to my son and to tell everyone how special he was to me."

After the memorial, a lunch was served. Elaine remembered, "Talking to friends and family at this time was very healing. To hear people's remembrances of Derek was painful, but it made me realize that Derek had touched so many people.

"One of the most painful experiences that day, other than knowing my son would never come back to me, was hearing comments like, 'Don't worry, you're both young. You'll have plenty of other babies.' Or, 'Derek's death was God's will, and you need to accept that.' After hearing so many of these painful comments, my uncle told me, 'Elaine, you may not know this now, but it is a good thing Derek died at three months rather than when he was older. The grief isn't as deep when you don't know your children.'

"My first reaction was seething anger. More than anything, I wanted to punch this old geezer. But before I let anything caustic slip from my mouth I remembered that my uncle had lost his two sons in a boating accident when they were in their late twenties. I looked in his eyes and saw his own grief and realized he thought he was comforting me. Still, it hurt me to think that others felt he wasn't yet a person; Derek certainly was. I loved him like I have loved nothing in this world. The suggestion that my grief was less than it would have been if he had died when he was older was ludicrous. I would have given anything I had to prolong his life by even another day."

After everyone left, Monte, Elaine, Jackie, and the couple's parents sat at a church table and reminisced about the beautiful boy that they had known for such a short time. Stories were told, memories captured, and tears were shed. As both sets of parents said their goodbyes, Jackie handed Elaine and Monte a frame. It was blue, and in it was a hand-calligraphied note that Jackie had written. It said:

Dear Mom & Dad,
I want you to have one last reminder of me. I know that you will never forget me, nor will I forget you. I will look forward to the day

when we can all be together again. But until that time I want you to know that I could not have asked for better parents. How goofy you are! Making me giggle all the time as you tickled my toes and kissed my nose. These memories I will hold dear, and I hope you keep them close to your heart too. I have met my siblings up here. They are beautiful, just like me. When you have grieved my loss and are ready to start your family again, they will come into your lives. I have taught them all about you. I have told them you love giggles and having your fingers held. I also told them they need to occasionally have a really messy diaper just to see your reaction. Take the time to miss me, but please go on with your lives. I will be watching you from on high. I am being well taken care of and I am caring for your other babies who will come. Please know my experience with you was the best thing in my short life.

Love,
Derek

As Elaine and Monte read the note, they both broke down in tears. This gift from Jackie was difficult for them to read through the flood of emotions, but it was a gift that would mean so much in the following months of recovery. Elaine remembered, "Of all the cards and notes, this one continues to be healing to me. I know that Jackie wrote it, but I like to think it was divinely inspired. I hung the frame in my living room, and there were many days I took it off the wall to read it. I would hold the frame next to me and hug it as I cried. It was my concrete remembrance of my son, and I thank God that I had it."

As the year passed, the couple hit many emotional highs and lows in their marriage. The lines of communication between them were down for a long time. They got through the days, but both were in shock, and they dealt with it differently. Monte remembered, "Elaine wanted to talk about his death all the time. It seemed pointless to me to rehash that pain; I couldn't do that. It hurt me to think about it all the time. For me it was better to move on, to try and keep it out of my mind."

Elaine attributed Monte's withdrawal to unhappiness with their marriage. She said, "I needed to talk to him about our loss, and he seemed so disinterested. One afternoon he was watching a ball game and I asked him if he would visit Derek's grave with me. He just looked at me and went back to watching his game. I sat on the couch and started sobbing, and he just lost control. He yelled at me and told me he was tired of seeing me cry all the time. That day we had the biggest fight we ever had. I told him I was unhappy and that I thought he had changed. I had loved his happy-go-lucky personality, but his personality seemed to have died with our son. This really seemed to be a turning point for us. It was almost as if we needed to say those ugly things to each other to wake us up from our dormant lives."

Monte and Elaine did not consciously decide when they would have another baby, but they did not use birth control after Derek's death. After two years without a pregnancy, Elaine began to worry. She didn't worry until then because with all of the stress and emotions related to Derek's death, she did not expect a pregnancy. But as life became more normal, she wondered why she hadn't conceived.

Elaine made an appointment with her general practitioner, Doctor A. The doctor did a papsmear and a pelvic, and told Elaine not to worry. He said that with all the stress she was going through, she probably wasn't ovulating. He prescribed the fertility drug, Clomid, and told her to take the drug on days five to nine of her cycle. He was so sure of his diagnosis that he did not even feel that temperature charting was necessary.

Elaine was frightened at the effect Clomid had on her body. She recalled, "I had been on Clomid for two days when the first hot flash hit me. I was in a meeting and all of a sudden I felt like I was burning up. Sweat started pouring off my face and I had to excuse myself to go to the ladies' room. When I got there I peeled off my jacket to find my shirt soaked with sweat. I ran cold water on my face, and the heat left as soon as it came. When I called my doctor, afraid that something was wrong with me, he treated me like a goof. He said that it was a side effect of the medicine and not to worry about it. I was so angry with him—not only did he not tell me that hot flashes could be a side effect, but he also treated me like a know-nothing blonde."

At that point, Elaine decided to take responsibility for being her own advocate in her medical care. She read about Clomid and found that the drug induces ovulation by stimulating the pituitary gland to produce hormones that start the ovulation process. Elaine also read about taking her basal body temperature to determine ovulation. Irritated that her doctor had not even told her about this, she bought a thermometer and took her temperature.

The first month on Clomid she did not become pregnant. For the next two cycles she discontinued Clomid so she could chart her temperature and see if she was ovulating. Her charts were like something out of a textbook: perfect twenty-eight day cycles with ovulation occurring on the fourteenth day. When she checked her cervical mucus it was clear and stringy, just the way it was described in the medical text she had referred to. From all indications, she was ovulating normally.

Armed with this information, she called her doctor to ask if it was still necessary for her to take Clomid. As she explained the situation, he told her that she really could not accurately diagnose ovulation from a chart. He advised her to take Clomid for three more months, and to come back if a pregnancy did not result.

Elaine was once again disgusted with her doctor's refusal to treat her with respect. After she hung up the phone, she called an infertility support group. Elaine remembered, "I knew I did not want to see Doctor A again; he was not treating the situation as if it were important. I looked in the yellow pages and found an infertility support group number. The copy said that they offered counseling and referrals. I called, and they gave me a few numbers of infertility specialists. When the woman on the line asked me how long I had been dealing with infertility, I informed her I wasn't infertile, and I hung up. Looking back on it, I suppose I knew there was a problem, but I wasn't ready to accept it at that point."

Accepting her infertility was a slow process. Elaine remembered, "I had gotten pregnant so easily before that I couldn't accept infertility as a diagnosis. I know now that secondary infertility is not uncommon, but I didn't know it then.

"My infertility started whispering its existence to me at odd times. Walking in a store and seeing a sign for maternity clothes, or watching television commercials that asked me if I thought I was pregnant; these were key factors in chipping away my assumption of fertility. I think I finally accepted my infertility when I saw a little baby who looked like Derek. I remember seeing him in a stroller and thinking he really resembled my son. Then I thought, *If only I could have another one.* I flinched at the realization that I had thought *if only.*"

Three months later, Elaine and Monte walked into a doctor's office. Elaine had elected to go to a reproductive endocrinologist, Doctor B. Monte remembered, "I was very nervous about seeing this doctor. I kept hoping we wouldn't have a problem, that somehow after examining Elaine the doctor would say, 'Infertility is not your problem, you are both fertile as ever.' The idea of losing our son and our fertility within such a short time was almost too much to bear."

This doctor met with the couple, asked about contraception use and Elaine's past gynecological history, and asked to see her temperature graphs. He then asked Monte if he had anything in his history that might affect his fertility. The doctor wanted to know if Monte had had mumps as an adult, had experienced a recent prostate infection, or if he was aware of whether his mother had taken the drug DES when she was carrying him. Monte told the doctor that none of those circumstances applied to him. After doing the pelvic exam, the doctor explained to the couple that he had felt a thickening of Elaine's tubes. He said that to be certain of the diagnosis, he would need to do a laparoscopy. He would also check to see if Elaine's tubes were open by running dye through the cervix. If the tubes were clear, the fluid would spill through freely. Elaine was scheduled for surgery for the next month, and Monte was advised to have a sperm analysis done.

Fear of the unknown can be a determining factor as to whether a couple will seek out treatment for infertility. Both Monte and Elaine had harbored deep fears about what would happen to them if they decided to seek medical advice and treatment, but they were glad they overcame them. Leaving the office after their initial visit, the couple felt some of their fears fade. The doctor had been gentle and reassuring with them. His concern had seemed genuine, and he had listened to their questions.

Monte's sperm analysis came back showing it was within the normal range. Monte said, "For me, it was such a relief to be told that we had at least one thing working in our favor. Although I never told Elaine, I was glad my sperm was okay. I felt I had disappointed her enough since Derek died—I'm not sure if I could have handled knowing I was the cause of our infertility."

Elaine spent the night before the laparoscopy in the bathroom, throwing up. She said, "I hate hospitals, and the idea of surgery, even a minor one, scared me to the bone. I kept trying to block out my fear, to pretend it didn't exist, but the pain in my stomach would not go away."

That night, Monte called Jackie and asked if she would come with them to the hospital the next day. She agreed to go. Jackie remembered, "Elaine was as white as a ghost. It was obvious how scared she was. I kept trying to make light of her situation, but she barely acknowledged my presence. When the nurse came to get her for surgery, Elaine grasped my hand and told me she didn't want to go. I didn't know what to say. I think I mumbled something about being strong and that we would see her in awhile." Monte helped Elaine into a wheelchair and the nurse brought her to surgery.

The procedure went smoothly, and while Elaine was in recovery, her doctor discussed his findings. He said that Elaine probably had had an infection that had occurred sometime after Derek was born, because the tubes were almost one hundred percent blocked. He explained that only a trickle of dye came out and that the lining of the tubes looked to be damaged. The options the doctor mentioned included another laproscopic surgery to open the tubes, and in vitro fertilization (IVF) to bypass the damaged tubes.

Elaine remembered, "As he talked, I kept thinking, *I don't want any more surgeries. I want this surgery to give me my baby.* The doctor explained that the surgical option would have had a better chance of helping me get pregnant if the tissue within my tubes wasn't so damaged. He said that the advantage of surgery over IVF would be that if surgery was successful, only one operation would be necessary. With IVF there would be a possibility that there would be many cycles to go through before ever achieving a pregnancy, if we did at all. He told me to recover and then think about our choices. If we were interested in finding out more about surgery or IVF, he said to contact him when we were ready. I began to sob, and as he left he patted my knee. I wanted to yell at him to come back and tell me everything was going to be all right."

Three months after the surgery, the couple met with the doctor and discussed their options. They elected to have a second surgery. The reasons they used to make their choice were cost, availability, and their financial resources. The couple realized that the cost for IVF could potentially be much higher than that for surgery. In order to have the IVF procedure done, Elaine would be put on medication that hyperstimulated her ovaries into producing as many eggs as possible. She would be monitored very regularly using ultrasound techniques. Then, when her follicles reached maturity, she would have to travel to another state to have the actual egg harvesting and transferring of embryos to the uterus done. The time and effort involved for this procedure was more than the couple were willing to concede. But the last and most decisive factor was that Elaine felt she could emotionally handle the surgery, but not the IVF. Elaine said, "When the doctor explained IVF, my red flags came up. He said they would transfer six living embryos to my uterus. After the death of my son, I felt that by transferring six embryos I would be condemning some of my children to death. I know to a lot of people it sounds ridiculous, but I had nightmares about more of my children dying."

The surgery was scheduled, and Elaine and Monte went home to wait. Monte remembered, "I never was very religious before my son died. After he died I was very angry, and I needed to vent my anger at someone; I decided that God was as good as anyone. For a long time I blamed Him for taking Derek. Sometime later, however, I found that my angry rantings had been replaced by my asking God to please take care of my son. I was surprised by how much comfort I felt after I prayed, and soon began to do it on a daily basis. To know that Derek was somewhere safe helped me live again. Before Elaine's second surgery, I prayed all the time. I asked God to guide us to a child—our child. I felt confident that He would help."

Elaine coped with her grief very differently than her husband did. Although she prayed, she found that the most comfort and relief came from being with children. After Elaine started seeing the reproductive endocrinologist, she volunteered to be a Big Sister. Her little sister was a seven-year-old girl named Tina. Elaine said, "At that time I felt an overwhelming need to parent, but to do so without full responsibility. Monte and I talked about becoming foster parents, but decided against it. Seeing a child come into our home only to leave again would be too much like the loss I felt with Derek. With Tina I was able to do things with her like a mother would. We went shopping, went to movies, and rode roller coasters like women possessed. Laughing with her and enjoying her youth made me feel good about myself again."

The day of the surgery, her parents, Monte, and Jackie accompanied Elaine to the hospital. Elaine's mood was in striking contrast to the one she had been in prior to her previous surgery. She joked with her family and the nurses, and generally seemed very relaxed. Monte and Elaine had prayed together the evening before and felt very optimistic about the chances of a pregnancy after the surgery. Monte said, "Praying together was something we had really never done before. It felt very good to be on the same wavelength as Elaine. We also felt that we knew a lot more going into this surgery than the previous one, and that really relaxed us."

Elaine was in surgery for about four and a half hours. Time passed very slowly for those who waited for her. The doctor finally arrived in the waiting room and talked with Monte. He said that the surgery went well, the tubes were cleared, but that the mucosal lining of the tubes looked to be in bad shape. The doctor said the only thing to do was to keep charting Elaine's temperature and to use an ovulation kit to time intercourse. Whether the surgery would help achieve a pregnancy, he could not say.

After Elaine woke up from the anesthesia, she was wheeled to her room. She was greeted by her family, bouquets of balloons and flowers, and cards. After a brief conversation with Elaine, Monte and her parents left her to rest for the evening. Jackie stayed behind and presented to her sister a little glass box wrapped with a red ribbon. Jackie told Elaine that she should open the box only if things looked as bad as they did after Derek died. Jackie explained to her sister that the note was a special "pick me-up" to be read only when she needed something happy in her life. Elaine remembered, "I was still kind of groggy, and thought Jackie's little box was kind of weird. But I thanked her and talked about how glad I was to have the surgery over with. The next day when I was released, I went home and I put the little box at the bottom of my underwear drawer, not thinking too much about it."

The first month after surgery, Elaine was positive that she would get pregnant. She felt that the past few years had been filled with darkness, and was looking forward to happier times. Elaine daydreamed about her new child and wondered how she would break the news of impending fatherhood to Monte. Monte, on the other hand, felt certain they would get pregnant, but was not laying odds on a pregnancy right away. After all, their first pregnancy had taken three months to happen.

Elaine dutifully took her temperature and used her ovulation kits. True to schedule, the kit indicated that Elaine would ovulate on the fourteenth day. By the twenty-seventh day, Elaine had gone out and purchased a pregnancy test, sure she was pregnant. The next morning her temperature had dropped, which indicated she was not pregnant, but she was desperate for a confirmation of a pregnancy and took the test anyway. Elaine remembered, "I knew I was pregnant. I didn't have the classic symptoms of pregnancy but I hadn't had them with Derek, either. When I saw my temperature was down I tricked myself into thinking I hadn't kept the thermometer in my mouth long enough. I jumped out of bed and took the test, and five agonizing minutes later saw that it was negative. I was stunned for a minute, and then I threw the kit at the bathroom mirror. I called in to work and said I wouldn't be coming in because I was sick. It was the truth—I was sick of my infertility, I was sick about the test being negative, and I was sick because my illusions had been taken from me. I cried the whole day, and nothing Monte said could comfort me."

As the months passed without a pregnancy, the couple's optimism was replaced by fear. They became more aware of their infertility each passing day. Elaine refused to go to the places she and Monte had once loved—no longer did they haunt the amusement park, the pool, the mall, or the lake, because these places were filled with parents and their children. Seeing these families laugh and enjoy themselves made the couple long for the days when they had their son with them. They felt like they were outsiders; they did not fit in with any group, and felt socially isolated. It became too painful to keep in close contact with friends with children, and friends who had no children by choice did not understand their pain. Monte and Elaine did not have friends who were infertile. So they withdrew to their house, feeling lonely and lost.

When the anniversary of her last surgery was two weeks away, Elaine called her doctor. She told him that she was not yet pregnant and wanted to know other options she could look into. Elaine remembered, "I was so desperate—I just kept asking him what we could do. He told me we could try IVF, but I told him that was not a viable option for us. He then said there were always the options of adoption or surrogacy. A few months before, Monte and I had contacted several state agencies concerning adoption. The agencies told us the waiting lists for babies were closed, and they did not think they would reopen for another few years.

"I cried as I asked him if there wasn't any other way, and he said that there really wasn't. I was just crushed. I really felt like we were at the end of the line."

It was at that point that Elaine called Jackie on the phone and wept as she recounted her conversation with her doctor. Jackie tried to comfort Elaine, and asked if she had ever opened the glass box. When Elaine answered no, Jackie told her to get off the phone and do it. Elaine said, "I was so devastated that I wondered how in the world a note in a glass box could make me feel any better. But Jackie was insistent, so I went and found it. I untied the ribbon and opened the box. Inside was a note." The note said:

Dear Elaine and Monte,

You are either reading this note because you are too curious or you are very depressed. In this note I am offering a gift to you. It is a gift that you must think very carefully about before accepting. But know that I will never ask for the gift back. If you accept it, it is yours forever.

I know that you have had surgery to try and become pregnant and that you are morally opposed to IVF. In all likelihood, you are not pregnant now. I would like to offer you a gift of an egg and a body to grow your baby inside of. Before you get too excited, know that I have thought about this for a long time. I have contacted a fertility specialist and she said I appear to be fertile. She said that if you were to choose this gift, I could be artificially inseminated using Monte's sperm, without too much effort on any of our parts. I have also contacted a lawyer and checked on the legalities of such a proposal. After the baby is born I will give the baby to you and you can adopt the baby as your own. No one will need to know about this. I assume you would want to tell Mom and Dad, but that is your choice. The only role I want in this is to be the baby's aunt. I will have biologically given this baby half of its genetic code, but you will be the child's mother from the moment it is conceived.

To see you in such pain has been incredibly difficult for me. I've always told you I would do anything for you. I hope you will consider accepting this gift.

Love,
Jackie

When Monte got home, Elaine was waiting for him at the door. She handed him the note and told him to read it. Monte remembered, "I couldn't believe what I was reading. It seemed like a dream—I was totally taken aback by Jackie's proposal. I looked at Elaine and I asked her what she thought, and she shrugged her shoulders. I read the note again, then folded it up. I changed the subject by asking Elaine what she wanted for dinner, and we didn't talk about the note again until a few weeks later. It was about twelve-thirty at night and we'd just shut the TV off. I turned to Elaine and told her that if she wanted to accept Jackie's gift that I would want to also."

Elaine said, "I told Monte that I wanted to be a mother more than anything, and if it meant that Jackie would carry the baby, I was for it. I hugged him and we called Jackie on the phone. Of course, we woke her up, but we couldn't wait any longer. We decided to meet the next day to talk with each other."

The three talked for a few months before any action was taken. To make such a monumental decision quickly would have been unfair to everyone involved. They reviewed medical procedures, legal matters, ethical considerations, and the possible consequences of surrogacy. Jackie said, "I told them over and over again that this baby would be theirs. At thirty-four I had no desire to get married or have a baby—that just wasn't part of my makeup. As a result, I felt that I was free to make that offer to them. If I had felt for a moment that I might renege, I would never have made the offer I did.

"As far as ethical considerations, they were never difficult for me to accept. My sister and I share our parents' genetic material. I was offering mine to my sister, and I never viewed this as giving my baby away. The thing that frightened me the most was wondering if this would hurt our relationship. I didn't want them to unconsciously feel that I was coveting their baby. I didn't want our relationship to end.

"Another issue that I was concerned about was making sure that their baby understood why he or she was born into this situation. I never wanted that child to feel that I did not love him or her. I would love that child as an aunt.

"If it would have been possible for my sister to accept the idea of IVF, using her eggs and having Monte and Elaine's embryos implanted in me,

I would have gone through that procedure. But I knew she could not accept that as an option."

For her part, Elaine said, "I wanted this to happen the very first time I read her letter. I was so unhappy and felt so depressed; I just didn't know how I was going to recover. Everything looked so bleak until I read about her gift.

"After we made the decision to go ahead with the surrogacy, I felt an incredible burden had been lifted from me. I would finally be able to parent another child—my child. That my sister could give me such a gift still astounds me. If the situation was reversed, I'm not sure that I could offer the same gift.

"I would never have looked for a surrogate mother. I would have been too afraid that the surrogate would want to keep the baby, and emotionally there was no way I could have handled that. If there was any part of me that questioned Jackie's decision, I would have declined immediately."

It took Monte a while longer to make the decision than it did Elaine. He said, "There were so many issues to consider. What would we tell our folks? What would we tell our friends? Was this an ethical choice? How would we tell our child of his or her background? How would Jackie treat me after the baby was born? How would Elaine view me if I accepted the gift? We talked about all those questions, and we made some hard decisions. Surrogacy was not a choice we made lightly. We researched it thoroughly and did a lot of soul-searching before we reached our answer.

"After we decided we would proceed with the surrogacy, I really became excited. The change in our attitudes toward life was amazing. It felt like my breathing wasn't restricted anymore, and I looked forward to becoming a father again."

Both sets of parents were told of the surrogacy plans. Although they found it shocking at first, the news was accepted by Elaine's parents. They knew the agony Elaine and Monte had been going through. Monte's parents, however, refused to accept the surrogacy or give their blessing. Monte recalled, "I knew before I told them that they were going to have a hard time with the concept of surrogacy, but I was shocked at how vehemently they were opposed to it. I remember my mother asking why we wouldn't consider IVF. After all, she asked, didn't we want to have 'our own' baby? Elaine jumped in and told her about her moral objection to IVF. And then my father said, "Don't you find it morally objectionable for someone else to get pregnant by our son?" Elaine started crying, and I told my parents that this was not their choice. I explained how painful it had been for us to experience Derek's death. By using IVF, we felt we would almost certainly have at least one more death on our hands. Elaine then stood up and said, 'Besides, it's not just anyone that's going to have our baby; it's my sister.' At that point we got up and left. The situation was so messy and so painful for us. It hurt me that my parents couldn't give us their blessing."

As a result of the disastrous meeting with his parents, Monte and Elaine held off on pursuing their surrogacy plans. Elaine recalled, "After that meeting, I felt so dirty. I was made to feel like I was some mad scientist trying to create an evil experiment; I was totally flattened. Monte and I talked once more about the ethics involved in a surrogacy agreement, and after a lot of discussion and even more tears, we decided our original decision was right for us. We wrote his parents a letter that told them our reasons behind our choice. We explained that we were sorry they objected to our decision, but that it was our decision to make. We went on to say that we hoped they could find a place in their hearts to accept our choice and the baby that would result from it. I included a poem that I had written after Derek's death to give them an inkling of how depressed and sad I had been. I told them that I needed a baby and would not apologize for that fact."

Soon after that, a contract was written between the couple and Jackie, and the first artificial insemination cycle began. Elaine remembered, "I was so excited—I felt like I was walking on air. I was surprised that I never felt sad or grieved that I would not be able to carry this child. I kept expecting to, but the feelings never came. I felt so lucky, so blessed that Jackie had given me the opportunity to be a mother again."

Jackie was inseminated three times before she achieved a pregnancy. Jackie said, "I knew I was pregnant about a week later, because I started having all the symptoms in the book. Every day Elaine would call and ask how I was feeling, and I'd say, 'Oh, just the same as usual,' even though I had just thrown up. I didn't want to get her hopes up before I was absolutely sure. The morning my period should have started was when I took the pregnancy test. It was positive, and I was ecstatic—my sister and her husband were going to be parents again. I thought about doing something cute to announce the pregnancy, but decided against it. I just went over to their house, walked in, and said, 'I'm pregnant.' I thought Elaine was going to jump out of her skin. They both came over and hugged me, and it was a very rewarding experience."

Two months after confirming the pregnancy, Jackie had her first prenatal checkup. Monte remembered, "We treated her like a fragile egg because she was holding the most precious gift of all. When they called her name, both Elaine and I trooped after her. I'm sure we got some looks from the people in the waiting room. After she was prepared for the ultrasound, we came and stood by her. The ultrasound technician said, 'Hey, Mom and Dad—you've got two babies in there!'

"Our emotions knew no bounds. Finally, after all the pain and frustration of infertility, we were free of that monkey on our backs. We were having twins. Two beautiful little heartbeats, two little lives sharing space together—those were our children. I thought my heart would burst.

"I hadn't seen or spoken to my parents since the big argument, so I decided to bring over the ultrasound picture of our babies for them to see. It was a very emotional scene. There was more heated discussion, and at one point I openly wept as I showed them their grandchildren's ultrasound picture. I don't think they had seen me cry since I was a boy. After that meeting, my parents began to loosen up, because they knew how important this was to me."

Elaine recalled, "After they said 'twins,' I didn't hear another word. I started jumping up and down. I could not contain my excitement, nor did I want to. Since I wasn't the one pregnant, the pregnancy had never felt real to me until I saw my babies on the ultrasound screen. I grabbed Jackie's arm and told her how excited I was, and she said, 'Yeah, I'd be excited too if it wasn't my stomach that was going to get stretch marks.' Then she laughed. I think she was scared and maybe overwhelmed, but I know she was happy for us."

The pregnancy was pleasantly uneventful. Elaine—and Monte, when he could—went with Jackie to all the prenatal medical visits. Jackie delivered the twins in the thirty-sixth week of her pregnancy. As she gave birth, Monte held one hand while Elaine held the other. Elaine remembered, "I kept telling her how much more fun this delivery was in comparison to Derek's birth. Jackie told me that she thought the other was one hundred percent easier.

"I can't describe the feelings I experienced when those babies came out. They were mine. They were beautiful. They were our life. After they got cleaned up, Jackie said hello to the babies. She said, 'Hi, kids, I'm your Aunt Jackie.' Jackie then asked us to each hold one of the babies while she rested. I held our daughter, Jacquelyn, and Monte held our son, John. Other than when I held Derek after he was born, I have never felt so complete than I did at that moment."

After Monte and Elaine brought the twins home, they decided that they weren't going to let them out of their sight. Elaine took a six-month sabbatical to stay home with her twins, and then Monte stayed with the children during the summer. For the first few months of their lives, Monte and Elaine checked their children's breathing every fifteen minutes. Elaine remembered, "We were so scared they were going to die. We overprotected them to the maximum. We didn't let them out of our sight, we kept them in the house most of the time, and we were always feeling their tummies to check their breathing. After the children lived past the age of Derek's death, I think we started to relax. We didn't talk about it very much, but the fear was always there in the back of our minds."

At the time of this writing, the twins are two years old. Monte, Elaine, and Jackie remain very close. The twins call Jackie 'Auntie Mom.' Since the day of their birth, the children have been told that Jackie carried them in her tummy and gave birth to them because Mommy wasn't able to do that. Jackie said, "The twins are such a blessing. They have made my sister and Monte happy again. The love I see in their eyes as they hold their children has made this experience unforgettable. If I had to do it all over again, I would make the same choice I did before. I have absolutely no regrets."

Through surrogacy, Elaine and Monte feel that they were given another opportunity to experience life as parents again. Their love and respect for Jackie is enormous. Monte said, "Jackie gave us our life back again. Elaine and I have finally put our marriage back on track. I changed after Derek's death, but now I find I am changing again. Losing our son and losing our fertility as a couple hurt us so deeply, but with that hurt came growth. We are a much stronger couple now because of what we had to deal with."

7

Deep inside of me is a piece of death.

It was supposed to be a new beginning.
It was a little dream waiting to happen.
It was alive, a bit scary,
and would mean big changes in our lives.

But now it is cold and lifeless;
no heat or rhythm could be found.
No more dreams can be dreamed.
No more, no more.

I cry. I cry all alone.
A few try to understand,
but try as they might
they do not feel the pain.

Life goes on for those around me.
But inside me, deep inside
is a piece of death.

Andrea wrote this poem after finding out, via ultrasound, that her baby's heart no longer beat. Two days later, her baby left her body in a pool of blood. This experience left Andrea shaken and numb. Shaken because she had loved that baby with every ounce of her being. Numb because this was at least her ninth miscarriage. She may have had more, but as the pain had taken its toll on her soul, she had stopped counting.

Alan and Andrea are in their thirties, have a successful marriage, and are the proud parents of three beautiful children. But in between the births of those children came the miscarriages. In medical terms, Andrea is diagnosed as a 'habitual aborter.' Her doctors did tests on her and autopsies on the babies, but they were unable to give Alan and Andrea any definitive reason why their babies kept dying. One doctor told them, "I think you just have been unlucky seven times."

Andrea's desire to have children started when she was a very young girl. She played with her dolls as though they were live, healthy children. She dreamed of being a real mom and wanted a dozen babies. When Alan thought of becoming a father, he fantasized himself as a wise and respected father and grandfather, one whom his children would look to for advice and love. They never questioned their ability to become parents, and both Alan and Andrea looked forward to starting their family.

Their first child was conceived a year after their wedding, and Alan and Andrea were elated with the news of impending parenthood. The pregnancy was healthy and uneventful, and in the month of December a beautiful, perfect son was born. There was never a concern about infertility, or about the ability to carry a baby to term.

A year later, Andrea realized that she was pregnant again. Since she had had an IUD inserted to delay having more children, she was very surprised about it. She went to her doctor to have her IUD removed, and even though the pregnancy was not planned, it was viewed by the couple as joyous gift. A month after the IUD had been removed, however, Andrea began to spot blood, and later miscarried the baby. Both Alan and Andrea felt sad, but they had not had a total emotional investment in the pregnancy. They felt that they were fertile and that the pregnancy had resulted in a miscarriage because of the IUD. When asked to describe her reaction to the miscarriage, Andrea said, "I was sure it was the IUD's fault and that I could get pregnant again very easily. I can remember thinking, *This is awful, but I can have another baby.* We weren't ready for a baby anyway."

After Andrea lost the baby, however, she started thinking about having more children. The baby's death had left a hole inside of her, and she felt the need to fill that empty feeling with another child. After discussing this with Alan, they decided to try and conceive another baby. It took a few months to conceive, and in that time Andrea grieved each cycle that did not result in a pregnancy. Each month Andrea was filled with excitement and anxiety as she looked forward to the new life that would grow inside of her. As the month progressed she became giddy with the idea of becoming a mother. At the end of the month, however, she was confronted with blood, the dark red substance that signified failure. When the bleeding started, the tiny sprig of hope died, and each period was the signal for Andrea to grieve.

Emotionally distraught and anxious, Andrea looked to Alan for solace, but found none. Alan could not fathom why Andrea was grieving, or why she was so pessimistic. Alan needed Andrea to be optimistic and Andrea needed Alan to grieve with her. Neither of their needs were met.

Months later, Alan and Andrea found out they were pregnant. Both felt happy and relieved. When Andrea was about two and a half months pregnant, she and Alan went camping with a few of their friends, over two hundred miles from their home. What was to have been a delightful, relaxing experience turned out to be a nightmare. Once they got there, Andrea discovered she had started to spot. There was a sinking feeling in her stomach as she discovered the dark red blood on her pants. Andrea remembered panicking and thinking the worst.

Alan rushed Andrea into the closest town. Away from their home town, away from their doctor, they had nowhere to turn. They found a doctor listed in the yellow pages. Their feelings of anxiety increased tenfold at having to go to a doctor who was a total stranger.

The medical office was shabby, cold, and sterile. The nurse instructed Andrea to undress and lie on the examining table, her feet in stirrups. An old country doctor walked in, and without introducing himself or asking for information, he began the pelvic exam. Afraid of the worst, Andrea lay shaking on the table. The doctor removed his fingers from her vagina and announced unemotionally, "Yep. You are going to lose it." He then walked out of the room. No comfort, no explanation, no instructions on what to do or to expect, absolutely nothing. As the doctor left, the nurse muttered an apology for the doctor's demeanor and then she, too, left.

Andrea remembered, "I asked Alan, 'Now what?' I got up and dressed, feeling like I had just awakened from a bad dream. We left and returned to the campgrounds and I remember thinking, *What's happening?*" Later, Andrea found a phone and called her own doctor. He told Andrea to not worry and let it bleed out, and to see him upon her arrival in town. Meanwhile, everyone was having a wonderful picnic. Andrea said, "I was sitting there trying to act as if nothing was wrong. My whole life had fallen apart, but I was supposed to go on."

Alan and Andrea told the others of the news, but there were no words of comfort or support for the couple. As a matter of fact, Alan himself believed that since there was nothing to be done about the miscarriage, they might as well enjoy the camping trip. Alan's way of dealing with grief at the time was to try and find the bright side of the situation.

Andrea said of the others' reaction, "It was like they thought I was just bleeding. After all, I was only two and one half months along—it was just a period. No big deal to them. No one said they were sorry. If anything, they left me off on my own, because they didn't know what to say, and they thought it was better to not say anything than to say something wrong. They just went on with the business of camping. It was a horrible weekend; I was so glad to have it over with."

When Andrea arrived home she again called her doctor, who repeated his advice to let it bleed out. She continued to bleed for three weeks. The doctor then told her that if she kept bleeding, they would need to do a D & C. Soon after that, however, the bleeding stopped. But as the blood stopped, her understanding of loss grew.

After this experience Andrea felt she had started an intimate relationship with grief. She said this relationship was hers alone: no one knew, and no one helped. She was sad and depressed and felt infuriated when people asked, "What's wrong?" Andrea said, "No one linked my emotions to this loss. The only one who acknowledged my baby's existence and grieved for it was me."

The days passed, but Andrea's longing for her baby did not. She was more determined than ever to get pregnant and carry her baby to term. Alan and Andrea tried for months to conceive a child, and each month a baby was not conceived felt like a personal failure for Andrea. The grief and desperation she felt mounted. Finally, Andrea became pregnant. She was elated and Alan was happy that his wife felt an emotion other than sadness. The pregnancy appeared to be healthy, and when the twelve week mark passed uneventfully, Andrea and Alan felt that this baby was destined to be born alive and healthy.

At sixteen weeks, Andrea woke up with incredible cramping. Frightened, she contacted her doctor with the news. He assured her that it was only nerves, and told her to relax. But Andrea told her doctor that she knew there was something terribly wrong. Again, her doctor dismissed her fears and said, "It's nothing. If it gets worse, come on in later this afternoon." Andrea remembered calling Alan at work and telling him the news. Wanting to comfort her, he suggested going to lunch together.

The cramping continued, however, and Andrea insisted Alan take her to the hospital that night. By eleven-thirty p.m. the cramps had turned into full-fledged contractions. Her doctor examined her and told them to go to the regional medical center, fifty miles away. In their shock, Alan and Andrea did not ask why the doctor had told them to drive in their own car instead of an ambulance. It was only on the way to the center that they began to think of the implications of their actions. What would happen if the labor kept progressing and Andrea started to hemorrhage? Alan drove close to ninety miles an hour on the interstate at midnight, trying to get to the medical center before the baby was born. On the way, Andrea kept reassuring herself that the doctors at the center would give her medication to stop the labor, and that her baby would be saved.

By the time they arrived at the emergency room, the amniotic fluid had broken, the baby was partially out, and Andrea was near hysteria. Her recollection of the experience was that of a cold, awful emergency room with interns and nurses coming in and out. She never saw the same staff person twice, and remembered thinking that she should charge admission to all of the gawkers coming into her room to watch. The care was mechanical and cold, never comforting. The contractions were intense, and Andrea did not want to push. For with each push, her baby inched closer to death.

As Andrea's labor progressed, Alan sat beside her and rubbed her arm, trying his best to calm and comfort her. Andrea was also surrounded by nurses who took her blood pressure and temperature, yet she still felt all alone. Alone in a sea of strangers, giving birth to a baby who would die.

Finally the baby came and the doctor caught it in a cold, silver dish. Too premature for any hope of survival, Alan and Andrea's baby died in an impersonal piece of medical equipment. Andrea felt the whole procedure was demeaning. She felt they treated her baby like it was nothing more than a glob of tissue in a bowl. She asked repeatedly to see and hold her baby, but the medical staff refused.

Andrea's cousin, Sheila, was a lab technician at the medical center. They asked for her, and she came in to see the couple. Andrea had told her cousin that she wanted to see the baby. Sheila talked to the attending staff and they finally brought Alan and Andrea's baby in for them to see. The baby was swaddled in a small towel. Andrea remembered, "The baby was tiny, with its head being bigger than the rest of the body. But it was perfect otherwise. It was the most perfect little figure I'd ever seen. And what I remember was being totally fascinated, not even sad at that moment. Just totally awed and fascinated by what I was holding and how far along it was." Andrea is a professor of Child Development. She remembered that as she studied her baby, she thought about her lectures on prenatal growth and development, and how her baby's appearance matched the information she gave her university students. The eyes were there but closed, the internal organs were starting to form, the male sex organs were there, the toes and fingers all there.

This was the first time during their infertility that Andrea saw Alan cry. Although this was Andrea's third miscarriage, it was the first time Alan openly grieved their loss. Andrea had resented the fact that Alan had not grieved with her before; that instead, he had only seemed to be moved by the fact that she had been sad and depressed. It was only when Alan showed remorse and grief at the loss of their son that some of Andrea's stored up rage at Alan dissipated.

For his part, it was only when Alan saw Andrea hold their son that he acknowledged that their loss was a human life. Alan admitted that he never bonded with the pregnancies the way that Andrea did. He did not spend a lot of time thinking about the fetus inside his wife as a living being. And as the earlier babies miscarried, he did not grieve the loss of a life, but only felt sad for his wife.

After they took the baby away, Sheila stayed with Andrea and Alan. They did not talk a lot, but Andrea remembered feeling very comforted by the presence of her cousin. That her cousin saw her pain and felt remorse made Andrea feel that finally somebody was there for her. As soon as Andrea was settled into a hospital room for the night, Alan left to take care of their young son. The rest of the evening was a blur to Andrea.

Her next recollection was waking up in the hospital room. She said, "Some dumb little nurse bopped into my room and asked me what I wanted to feed my baby. And I had to tell her my baby was dead. The horror of having to do that—I just cried for hours. I felt like telling someone 'Can't you even be sensitive enough to keep these idiots out of my room?' They had me right in the midst of all these new mothers. They were all having their babies brought to them to nurse. And there I was without a baby. Then I walked around to the intensive care nursery and looked at all the preemies."

Even if they survive, extremely premature babies often have very severe physical and mental disabilities. Life for these babies can be short and filled with pain and suffering. As much as she wanted her baby, Andrea did not wish that fate for her child. "I thought that if the baby had been older and lived, it would have been there, and that would have been horrible and nightmarish."

Among the experiences imprinted on her mind, Andrea will never forget her treatment by one of the doctors. He had not been there the previous night, but was assigned to her for the following day. She remembered thinking that he was one of the coldest, most insensitive medical professionals she had ever dealt with. His care was sterile and mechanical. Andrea did not remember any specific thing he did wrong, but had a general sense that this well-respected gynecologist was totally unfeeling.

Andrea now believes that her experience with this miscarriage was much more traumatic than it needed to be. She feels that medical staff need to be trained in appropriate bedside manner when it comes to miscarriages. A kind word, some show of support, and tenderness are invaluable in helping a couple's healing process begin. Andrea knows she will never forget her baby's face, but wishes she could have had a picture taken of her son as a concrete remembrance. The biggest regret Andrea has was not insisting on taking the baby home to bury it. The medical staff urged her to let them use the baby as a lab specimen. Weeks later, she received a lab report stating that the baby she lost was a perfectly formed male fetus.

The next day Alan went to work, and picked Andrea up at the hospital on his way home. It hurt Andrea that he had gone instead of spending the day with her. Miscarriages, especially those that occur late, can be devastating. Andrea felt that she had been left to fend for herself, lying in a hospital bed, bleeding, weak, and grieving her son's death. When Alan arrived, there was little communication about their loss. He desperately wanted Andrea to feel better, so he suggested they tour the city's waterfalls before going home. Andrea remembered, "I was thinking, *I could care less about them. I'm so tired and weak; why are we doing this?* I think it was something Alan was doing to try to help me, but it didn't. It was an attempt, and I think he thought it would be comforting, but it certainly wasn't. Yet I knew he was trying, so I didn't tell him I didn't want to go."

Learning to engage in open and healing communication was a continuing problem for Alan and Andrea as they attempted to overcome their tragedies. Andrea said, "I tried to talk to him and he just wasn't open. If I'd talk about how empty I felt, his responses to me included: 'We can try again in a little bit,' and 'We've got one child—be grateful for that.' It didn't take many of those responses before I realized it was a closed book. I felt like I was allowed a week to grieve before I was told to get on with it and to cheer up." It took Alan a couple of years before he realized that trying to be optimistic and expecting his wife to be also was an unsuccessful tactic. Alan said, "I've always been optimistic, tried to look on the bright side of things, but I've found out that doesn't work in this situation. I've tried to change this response, but it's something that I'm still working on."

Of the experience, Andrea said, "What I needed to do was bury that baby and have a funeral. To have officially acknowledged and grieved for that baby would have been healing. I also wish I would have given my baby a name." Andrea has talked with her minister and told him how important it is for a couple who have had a miscarriage to have a funeral or memorial service for their lost child, no matter how far along that child was in its development. Andrea believes a service acknowledges the child that died and how important the baby was to the family. Both she and Alan believe that a miscarriage needs formal closure for the family to heal.

The horror of losing the baby was magnified for Andrea after she got home. A few days following her return, her in-laws had a family gathering at their farm. Andrea talked to all of her relatives, and although they all knew about it, no one mentioned her miscarriage. Andrea almost wondered if she had actually had a miscarriage, because everyone acted as if nothing had happened. No one talked about it, no one asked how she was doing, no one said they were sorry. There was no acknowledgement that Andrea had been pregnant, nor of the fact that her beautiful, tiny son was now dead. Andrea's agony was compounded by the silence. She felt she was being told to suffer the pain in private and not complain.

After three miscarriages, Andrea desperately needed to gain some insight and perspective on past events. She remembered going to the library and to bookstores trying to find a book that would validate her experiences. For a long time she found nothing. Then one day she found a book, and devoured the information. She brought it home and asked Alan to read it. Andrea said, "I don't think he ever did. He just wasn't at the point of needing it. I wanted so desperately for him to understand what I was going through, but he didn't. He just deals with life so differently. For Alan, the pregnancies weren't real—he wasn't experiencing them. I don't even think that our three children were real to him until after they were born. Then he came alive and became an active participant. The fact that he didn't share grief with me is a scar that I don't think will ever heal."

Realizing that she needed to share the pain with someone, Andrea became more open to friends. She recalled, "I had a really good friend who had had a miscarriage. One of the things she gave to me was a little doily with a crystal prism in the middle. She said, 'No one else in the world will remember your baby—but you and I will. And we will know that the little prism is that spark of life that died, and that we still remember.' Her gift was such a comfort. Most of the words and gifts that have comforted me have come from someone who has experienced miscarriage too."

Andrea feels that women and couples can benefit immensely by sharing their pain with others who have had similar experiences. Being able to share the pain and grief without having to explain it is healing in itself; there is great comfort in knowing that one is not alone. Andrea also recommends that couples always tell someone that they are pregnant early on. Alan and Andrea found that telling someone about the pregnancy meant that if the baby died, someone else knew about its life. If they told, they weren't alone with their grief.

Some time after the third miscarriage, Alan and Andrea decided to pursue adoption, never doubting the old adage of 'You can always adopt.' They hit dead end after dead end. Andrea said, "It was the most hopeless thing I'd ever tried. We'd call social service agencies and find out they had a two year waiting list—we couldn't even get on those. I tried to get addresses of agencies that dealt with international adoptions, and it seemed there were still no babies. We just couldn't get on anybody's waiting lists."

People would tell Andrea that even though she couldn't adopt, she should be grateful for the child she already had. What those people did not understand was that Andrea and Alan were grateful for their child, but it did not take away the desire for another baby. Having a child did not make the black hole in Andrea's soul go away.

A few months passed, and Andrea attempted to get her life back on track. One evening her cousin Sheila knocked on her door. Andrea remembered thinking the visit odd, because the two women weren't in the habit of visiting each other. Sheila asked Andrea to take a walk with her. During the walk Sheila told Andrea that she would be willing to carry a baby for Andrea and Alan—to be a surrogate mother. Sheila said she had decided to make the offer because she had witnessed the pain and despair the couple went through when they lost their son. Sheila felt that by offering to be a surrogate, she could help Alan and Andrea to overcome their grief and restore some joy to their lives.

Andrea was touched and moved by Sheila's offer. Here was someone who wanted desperately to reach out and help her, and she marvelled at Sheila's selflessness. Andrea and Alan explored the issue for a long time. After much discussion, however, the couple decided that Sheila would be making too huge a sacrifice. A baby would be wonderful, but they felt it would be unfair to Sheila and her parents. The decision was made, and Sheila was told of it. For Andrea, the decision was painful, but the thought behind her cousin's gesture would never be forgotten.

During this time, Andrea and Alan were still trying to conceive, and each month that passed without a pregnancy became increasingly traumatic for Andrea. There was no support for her despair over her infertility. Each time she tried to talk to her husband about her feelings of desperation and loss, he suggested they stop trying to have any more children. But while Andrea had difficulty dealing with the emotions brought on by her infertility and miscarriages, what her husband suggested was not even remotely possible for her. She tried talking to her mother, Lyla, but every time Lyla was confronted with Andrea's pain, she backed away.

Finally, Andrea decided to seek professional help in trying to achieve and maintain a pregnancy. She went to an endocrinologist, and he did an infertility workup. He diagnosed a hormone problem and prescribed the fertility drug, Clomid.

Andrea's first month on Clomid resulted in a pregnancy. She was joyous, but afraid for her baby's life. Her doctor recommended progesterone shots twice weekly. In order to keep her pregnancy viable, Andrea would drive one hundred miles twice a week for sixteen weeks to get her shots. In addition to the progesterone shots, there were also many tests and much lab work required. Andrea went to most of these appointments alone, and once again, she felt abandoned in her quest to have a healthy baby.

During this time her university students complained that she looked tired and appeared to be unenthusiastic. Andrea remembered thinking that she was doing the best she could under the circumstances. None of them knew what she was going through, but their words and accusations stung her deeply.

Four and a half months into the pregnancy, Andrea tested positive to high blood sugars. She had pregnancy-induced diabetes, and ended up requiring insulin shots and needing very careful monitoring for her high-risk pregnancy. Andrea remembered, "The whole pregnancy was so scary. I feared the worst all the time." As it turned out, Andrea delivered a baby boy via a caesarean section in September of 1982. Her son was healthy, beautiful, and perfect in every respect.

This baby meant the world to Andrea. For the first half hour of his life he lay on a warming table next to his mother. She was not allowed to hold him until the doctors checked his condition thoroughly to assure he was healthy. Andrea remembered, "I couldn't hold him, but he held my finger for the first half hour of his life. Lying next to my son was incredibly life-affirming. My thoughts were that I never wanted to leave him. If I could have sat and rocked him in my arms for the rest of my life, I would have."

Finally, the couple had a healthy baby to love and rejoice over. The celebration, however, was dampened by the death of Alan's grandmother the day before their son's birth. Alan was there for the birth, but then had to leave to be a pall bearer at his grandmother's funeral. His parents were in shock, and their grief did not leave much room for their new grandson. Andrea said, "They were spending all of their time going through the belongings—Alan's dad never came down to see his grandson, and his mom came for maybe fifteen minutes and spent the whole time talking about what she was going to inherit. She didn't even look at the baby, and it just hurt. For his first seven years it was like they hardly knew the kid existed, because they had never bonded to him."

To compound the situation, Lyla's husband had checked into the hospital the same day Andrea checked in to have her baby. They found out that he had cancer. Andrea remembered, "They were in the process of dealing with his cancer, and it seemed like I worked forever to have this beautiful baby and nobody cared. It was like nobody had time to enjoy this wonderful gift. I think that hurt almost as bad as the miscarriages.

"I kept thinking that if it had been a girl, my mom would have been excited about it. But that's not fair of me. She was going through her own hell and stress, but at the same time I had wanted this baby so badly and nobody celebrated with me when he was born. My mom attached to him quickly later on; it just wasn't what I expected. Then my sister Rhonda had a baby girl the next year, and of course by then, my mom was all excited. Soon after, I found out I was pregnant again, and I miscarried weeks later. I didn't even tell anyone I was pregnant, so again, I grieved alone. Then Alan's sister Meg had a daughter, and his mother went down to be with her, buying the baby all sorts of gifts. That brought back all the hurt from lack of attention that had been given to my son. There was such a feeling of jealousy when other people were having their babies. And Alan would say, 'You should feel good for them, you shouldn't feel jealous of them. You should feel happy for them.' But that just wasn't part of my makeup."

A few months later, Andrea found out she was pregnant again. She went down to her doctor and took a test which confirmed her pregnancy. To celebrate, Andrea bought a tiny music box for her baby. As she got out of the car, however, the music box fell to the ground, smashing on the sidewalk. Andrea began to cry. She had bought this gift for her baby, and it had broken—Andrea wondered out loud whether this was an omen of things to come.

A week later, Andrea started spotting and had another blood test. The test showed her hormone levels had gone down instead of up, and her doctor recommended an immediate D & C. Her mother and children were with her; they had no indication this would turn into an emergency situation. Andrea said of the experience, "Before I knew it I was down in surgery having a D & C. And then it was over with, and we went back home. I got home tired, weak, and emotionally drained, and Alan left me at home with the boys so he could go to a meeting.

"I felt so totally unloved; I thought that if I were pretty, if I were someone wonderful, he would care for me. But since I was the old horse around the home—the old rag that hangs around the house—I might as well take care of the kids. I remember feeling like I once again wasn't going to get any support from Alan. Suffer in peace, it was no big deal, and get back to life as usual. So that's what I did. Feeling empty, feeling like a failure, feeling unloved."

Four weeks later, Andrea woke up with terrible cramping. While sitting on the toilet she felt a strange sensation, and she cupped her hands underneath her and caught a bloody sack. She realized she had lost yet another baby. Putting the remains in a baggy, she and Alan went to see her doctor. The doctor examined her and advised another D & C. The only thing Andrea remembered thinking was not wanting to go through the process yet again. She did not want to go under the anesthesia, and felt unemotional about the loss of the baby because she was so emotionally exhausted.

The reports from the lab stated that the expelled fetus had been in gestation eight weeks and had spinabifida. About the report, Andrea said, "Sure it did—they had scraped it four weeks earlier with the last D & C. I lost faith in the doctor. He had no explanation—he didn't even want to attempt to explain it. In fact, from that point on the doctor tried to avoid me. He wouldn't even make appointments.

"Sometime later I got pregnant again, and he wouldn't even see me. He referred me to a high-risk specialist. It was like he had washed his hands of me, like he didn't want to deal with somebody so awful and so complicated. He didn't have any answers, and so he didn't want to have to deal with me. It got to the point that I couldn't think about what had happened because what came to mind was what might have happened if

I hadn't had the first D & C. Would I have a live, healthy baby now?"

Andrea did switch over to a high-risk specialist, and she was glad she did. He was an incredibly warm, supportive doctor. He treated her like a person, and seemed capable of understanding what had happened to her. He genuinely wanted to find answers for the couple. In fact, Andrea felt like they were searching for answers together. He encouraged questions and responded to them without hesitation. Both Andrea and Alan felt they were active decision makers with this doctor, which was something they desperately needed. When dealing with infertility and repeated miscarriages, control becomes an important issue to many couples. Finding a doctor that respects and involves patients in their medical care is vital to patients' emotional survival.

Alan and Andrea worked with this specialist and became pregnant again. A few months later they decided to visit friends who lived out of state. The first stop on their trip seemed uneventful. They went to dinner, but soon after eating, Andrea began feeling ill. Driving from the restaurant, Andrea had Alan stop the car so she could throw up. By the time they got to their friend's house later that night, she felt very ill. Andrea went to bed, but in the middle of the night roused Alan to take her to a hospital. The pain and fear she was feeling intermingled, and Andrea dreaded finding out what was wrong with her.

Andrea was admitted to a hospital where an ultrasound was performed to check on the pregnancy. The doctor told her the baby was no longer living. They put her in a room and she miscarried the baby while sitting on the toilet, almost passing out. Alan left to spend the night in a hotel, and the next morning he came to pick her up. Andrea remembered, "I was so weak and tired; I didn't want to check out. I felt so unimportant. I wasn't even worthy of a day to recover in the hospital. I had to get up and get on with my life—after all, tomorrow is a new day! I wasn't even allowed to grieve. I had to go back to our friends and continue our visit. I had to take care of my two noisy, active boys on a very long trip. I had no time to be weak or sad." Andrea was very angry with Alan for his response to her grief. She felt he had no understanding of what she needed, and her self-esteem was so low that she couldn't honestly say at the time if her needs were as important as she thought.

A few months later, Andrea miscarried another baby soon after she found out she was pregnant. There wasn't time to get excited about the pregnancy, or scared. The baby was there, and just as suddenly, was gone. For Andrea, it was just one more blow to her battered sense of self-worth.

The next miscarriage Andrea had was to be the most emotionally draining of all. She was about two months pregnant when a new concern crowded out everything else. Her husband Alan had found a lump on the side of his neck which was diagnosed as a fast-growing lymphoma, a cancer similar to Hodgkin's disease. His doctors sent him out of state for treatment. By the time they reached the medical center, Andrea was feeling very ill and had started to spot. She was so emotionally drained from dealing with her husband's cancer, however, that the bleeding was just one more awful event. Andrea recalled, "I called my doctor and he said, 'Just do what you can. If you need to talk with doctors there, go ahead.' For the first two days there we felt like we were cows being herded from one area to the next. And my thoughts were that it didn't matter—what I had to do was tend to Alan and give him emotional support. I just dealt with it as a horrible cramp day—I knew the baby was a goner and I couldn't deal with it. And I wasn't sure I should be pregnant anyway; I thought my husband was about to die."

The couple checked Alan into the hospital that evening, and he was scheduled for surgery in the morning. Andrea went back to the hotel alone and started to hemorrhage. She passed out on the bed and awoke later in a pool of blood, too exhausted to call for help. She said, "I think I didn't care to call for help. I think I was too depressed, too alone, too stressed out. By morning the bleeding had lessened and I knew I wasn't going to die or anything."

Andrea went to the hospital for Alan's surgery. The doctor came in and informed the couple that the cancer had spread to Alan's kidneys as well. He went on to say that Alan's lymphoma was not stage one cancer as originally thought, but stage four.

Soon after getting this news, Andrea's mother and pastor came to offer support to Alan. Andrea remembered, "The minister must have gone back (to my home town) and talked about how I was suffering both the cancer and a miscarriage at the same time, because we must have gotten hundreds of cards from the church during the next couple of weeks. I remember thinking, *Geeze, I never remember to send people cards.* I just hung on to every single one of them. Those cards are what got me through each day. They wrote not only about the cancer, but about the miscarriage as well. It was like they cared about me, too!

"Even through the cancer I would get really jealous of the attention my husband would get. I would think, *Damn, look at all the times I have been in pain and sorrow and nobody cared.* But Alan had an illness, you see. And I'm thinking, *I went through hell too. If you only knew what hell I went through.* So I had mixed emotions, feeling equally forlorn and lost about him and jealous of all the attention he got. I went with Alan to all his appointments, and his mom would come along. And I thought, *Where were you guys when I was going through all my hell?*"

Before Alan was released he had one more appointment with his doctor. Alan had realized that Andrea had been going through an incredibly difficult ordeal between his cancer and the miscarriage, so he asked his doctors about the possibility of having children in the future. The doctor told him he could bank sperm to use in the future. They didn't know what chemotherapy would do to sperm, but Alan could become sterile after treatment. However, banking sperm usually takes a few weeks to get enough usable specimens, and Alan did not have that time—the cancer was fast-moving, and aggressive treatment needed to start immediately.

Andrea said, "We thought about the dilemma of what to do. Was it really that important? After all, we had two healthy kids. Why worry about another one? But for once, it was Alan who said we needed to do it. I was ready to say, 'No, let's start the chemotherapy,' but Alan wanted to bank the sperm first."

Alan and Andrea found out there was a bank that would take the sperm and freeze it if the sample got to them in time. The sperm would remain viable for only a matter of hours, and Alan had to wait a day in between gathering samples to build up his sperm count. Each time the couple would box the sample up, put it on ice, and send it off. The bank would pick it up at the airport and transport it to the facility to be frozen. Alan and Andrea bought a plane ticket for each sperm sample. Andrea remembered, "It had to be like clockwork. I don't care what meeting we were in—we would watch the clock and then leave, because we knew what time the plane took off. We would rush home and somehow have to get this sample, and it was like, can you do it on command? Somehow we would have to figure out how to get relaxed enough to get this sperm, knowing that time was running short. One time we were rushing to get the sample and our youngest son walked in and said, 'Whatcha doing?' We referred to the samples as 'Joe Junior,' and we got to the point where we would just laugh about it. But it was really serious, and I couldn't believe how much emotional insurance it gave me. Alan was wise to do it, because that hole of emptiness was still there after I got over the shock of his cancer. That need for the baby was still there."

Andrea and Alan had to make some hard decisions about their lives. They had a lot of legal issues to contend with, and so they wrote a will which provided instructions for what would be done with the sperm samples, among other things. Andrea also decided that she would go to graduate school to obtain her doctorate degree. She felt that if her husband were to die, she would need the degree to support her two boys. After Alan's chemotherapy treatments ended, however, his follow-up tests indicated that he was cancer-free. The whole family felt an enormous weight lifted from its shoulders. They began to feel a sense of control coming back into their lives.

In her second semester of graduate school, Andrea once again found out she was pregnant, and for the first time, she did not want to be. She was taking care of her boys, worrying about her husband, and trying to complete grueling course work. Andrea felt she did not have the time or the energy to devote to the pregnancy, but she lost the baby before she had much time to contemplate what was happening. Andrea said of the experience, "I dealt with the miscarriage. It was a two-week pain period; I had had so many miscarriages that I had learned not to hurt so much. I also recovered quicker because I had never let myself get too emotionally involved in the first place. I had been so numbed from the previous experiences—I'd been through so much horror that I simply couldn't get as emotionally involved. I wouldn't let myself." Andrea lost the baby, but realized that chemotherapy had not left Alan sterile after all.

Although Andrea had not planned the pregnancy and had seemed to recover quickly, it left a gaping wound in her soul. The need for a live baby was stronger than ever. Andrea once again looked into adoption. She called the state social service agency, Lutheran social services, and Catholic social services. Andrea remembered talking to a nun and asking if it was possible to get on a waiting list for a baby. The nun told her there were no available openings. Andrea became distraught and cried on the phone, asking what was left for her to do. The nun told her to not lose hope. Although she had heard this before, the nun's words were comforting to Andrea. Later that summer, she found herself pregnant. Andrea believes the nun had special pull with God, because this pregnancy resulted in a beautiful daughter.

Andrea wanted this baby to live with every fiber of her being. She tried to stay as optimistic as possible. Excited about her pregnancy, she told her mother the news. Andrea remembered, "When I told my mother, she said, 'Oh, how awful!' I wanted to slug her. I hated her attitude." In retrospect, Andrea realized that her mother's response came from the fear that Andrea would be devastated by a miscarriage once again. At the same time, however, Andrea did not interpret the statement that way, and she still believes this is a scar that will never vanish. Her mother's statement epitomized the lack of support Andrea felt.

Andrea again went to a high risk specialist. She was elated to see her baby's heartbeat at six weeks. There were many tests to chart her baby's progress. The test results indicated she did not need progesterone shots and did not have diabetes, and the amniocentesis results showed a beautiful, healthy baby girl was growing inside of her. Andrea was incredibly tense through the entire nine months, but the pregnancy remained viable. Her daughter, Angel, was born in April of 1989.

During the pregnancy, Andrea had felt like she was on pins and needles; hoping for the best, but fearing disappointment and anguish. One of the ways she alleviated some of her fears and anxiety was by writing. In her third trimester she wrote the following letter to her baby:

Dear Tikki,

How slow the weeks seem to go as I wait for your birth. I'd give anything if next week was April instead of February. I'm so scared. I don't want anything to happen to you. I long to hold you in my arms and know that you are alive, well, and healthy. You will be spoiled. I plan to give you the very best that money can buy. I can't wait to buy you toys, kitchen sets, dolls and other things—even boy toys if you want.

I should be studying, working on my Ph.D. degree. But you know I don't care about it at all. I only seem to be interested in how you are, what you will be like. I've waited a long time for you. I pray, I beg God that you will be all right!

I would like to be able to nurse you, but I don't know if I can. It never worked for your brothers. But I will try. I can't wait to fix up your room. I hope you like pink and dainty things. I can't wait for you.

Andrea also began to use writing to document her pain and to help her accept loss. Two years later she wrote this poem to acknowledge and grieve for her last miscarriage:

> *Little pink bear*
> *you were for Katie Jo.*
> *But she will never be.*
> *I guess you will have*
> *to stay here with me.*
> *Together we will dream*
> *of what might have been.*
> *The hugs we might have had.*
> *I'll give you my love*
> *if you help me deal with my loss.*
> *Through you maybe Katie Jo can live.*
> *At least in my heart and my mind.*

Friends and relatives had witnessed the devastation Andrea experienced from her miscarriages. Their questions had included, "Why continue?" "Why purposely get pregnant?" and "Why is she putting herself and her family through such torment?" In answer to those questions, Andrea said, "To me, to not try meant there was no hope. The pain of not having hope was by far more painful than a miscarriage. Emotionally, I had no choice but to keep trying. Every one of my pregnancies had hope, even if the baby died." She advises couples to keep trying to reach their dreams and to avoid people who are negative.

Andrea has experienced more torment in eighteen years than most people experience in a lifetime. When asked how she survived her personal tragedies, she answered, "God has made me strong. He has always been an important part of my life. That's not to say I have always kept my faith. I have questioned, bribed, and threatened God. I questioned His existence, I wondered if He loved me, I hated Him for letting me experience all this pain in my life. For a time there were periods that I had a hard time at church. I went, but I couldn't sing, and I couldn't do the liturgy. Still, I always went—I could not leave totally. I did everything wrong with God, but He always pulled me back. He may not have answered my prayers the way that I asked, but He always answered. He didn't always give me my baby, but He gave me ways to cope. I know He does not cause the pain; instead He gives us ways to help us cope. I've learned He does intervene, He does save lives, and He is always there for us if we choose to let Him into our hearts."

Alan and Andrea's tragic miscarriages have ended at the time of this writing. Alan has been cancer-free since 1987 and continues to have a very positive attitude about his health. Andrea has been advised to have her tubes tied, and she feels that she probably needs a hysterectomy because of pain and excess bleeding. Still, she admits that she cannot consciously close this door on her life, and that it is hard for her to take the step that will mean she will not have another child. The longing for a baby will never leave Andrea, and she suspects that the first thing she will do when she dies is to go to heaven and hug each and every baby she has lost. It will only be then that the emptiness in her soul will be completely filled.

RESOLUTIONS
Surviving Infertility

In writing this book and interviewing individuals, I have learned a lot about myself, my husband, Duane, and the complexity of infertility. Those interviewed for this book have lived through the devastation of infertility and have found ways to cope and heal. As I recorded their stories and witnessed their grief, I began to better understand it, as well as my own struggles with infertility.

The same concerns and issues kept reappearing as I interviewed the families. I grieved that so many of us had felt we were all alone in our infertility, when in reality there were so many of us. I cried with the realization that we had needed to read a book like this when we were in the middle of hurting and had had none. We needed to witness others' grief as a way for us to see we weren't alone. Perhaps if we could have been able to do this early on in our infertility we could have had fewer lonely, isolated nights; we could have realized that the feelings we felt were not abnormal; we possibly could have been spared some of the depression that eventually led to thoughts of suicide or divorce; and we might have found the strength to survive the adversity of infertility a little earlier in our lives.

Everyone in this book who has been affected by the curse of infertility has had to develop coping mechanisms to deal with the heartache, humiliation, misunderstandings, and frustrations that haunt them every day of their lives. This concluding chapter examines infertile individuals' ideas on how to survive infertility, and is also meant as a guide for others to use when dealing with those struggling with infertility.

IF YOU ARE TO SURVIVE INFERTILITY YOU MUST:

➤ Learn to become an emotionally strong person. When you start infertility treatments you may not be, but you must learn to become strong if you are to endure the pain, frustration, and disappointments that are involved with infertility. Be aware that friends and relatives you count on for support may not understand your problem, and may unintentionally hurt you with their comments and actions. Be aware that not all medical professionals will be able to give equal attention to your emotional needs as they work to help you overcome infertility.

➤ Go into treatments with an open mind and learn to roll with the punches. As you work towards finding answers to your problem, you will need to discard old ideas, values, and philosophies. To endure infertility, you cannot come into it with a fixed set of ideas of what you will and will not do. If you decide on a course of action, and that you will not deviate from that plan before you start the race, you likely won't finish it. Dealing with infertility requires adaptability. You must keep an open mind in order to deal with it.

Andrea, who went through many ordeals in her attempts to have children, said, "I met a woman the other day. She had just realized she has a fertility problem, and she told me that she would take Clomid. But if she wasn't pregnant in three months, that would be it—she didn't want to be one of those women who became totally obsessed by a baby. My guess is that in three months she may very well be singing a new tune."

➤ Become an advocate for your own medical care. Research infertility and current treatments so you are aware of what could be the problem. Once you have done this, find a specialist who fits your needs. If you are unsure of where to look for a specialist, ask infertile friends or acquaintances where they go, contact your local hospital or community referral service, or contact *Resolve,* a national organization for people dealing with infertility (it is listed in the Resources section that follows this chapter).

Every individual has different needs, and one kind of specialist cannot meet the needs of everyone. Meet with at least two different doctors before you initiate treatment, so you can make an informed decision. Characteristics of a good specialist include: specialized training in infertility;

an aggressive commitment to helping find answers; a willingness to explain procedures, techniques, and costs; a helpful and caring staff; availability during evenings, weekends, or holidays for infertility treatments; a desire to help patients become involved decision makers; and a sincere and appropriate bedside manner.

When Sara first sought infertility treatment, she relied on a recommendation from a friend. "My friend Liz had been seeing a specialist and she raved about his abilities. I needed to see someone, so I went to him. I found him to have absolutely no bedside manner, and I couldn't imagine coming to see him week in and week out, trying to explain my lack of cervical mucus or to relay feelings of inadequacy."

➤ Realize that infertility treatments can be humiliating and degrading. Preparing for this fact can help you to see past the embarrassment to the possible results.

Lois, who has been struggling with infertility for years, told me, "When I got married I was so prudish I never even dreamed of mentioning to my husband that I even had a period. After a few infertility treatments, however, I kissed modesty goodbye. It was a burden, and when I disposed of it, I felt empowered to try any treatment."

➤ Keep the lines of communication open with your spouse. This is a vital component not only to dealing with infertility, but also to keeping your marriage viable. The stressors of infertility are incredibly demanding. It is important to talk to each other early on about expectations, feelings, methods of grieving, and treatment options. Sometimes this is not easy to do, but keep trying to listen to each other. It is very easy to get to a point where you stop talking altogether, and once that point is reached, it is very difficult to survive infertility.

Pete, a man who spoke at a recent meeting of a support group, pointed out just how difficult that can be. "Karla and I did pretty well until they found that I was the cause of infertility in our marriage. That hit me like a ton of bricks. When I thought Karla was the cause, I talked to her all the time and let her know that I was always behind her. We had a lot of late night talks, and I would leave little supportive notes around the house when her cycle started. But then it was my fault, and I found myself constructing walls, and I stopped talking. Karla kept at me, though, and I was finally able to share with her my feelings of depression and inadequacy."

➤ Respect your mate's feelings. It is important to understand that there may be procedures or treatments that your spouse fears or is opposed to. Let your spouse know your reaction, but make sure to respect his or her feelings. Do not try to force your spouse into changing his or her mind. Instead, examine your feelings and communicate about possible options.

Lisa and Bill disagree on what treatments are acceptable. Lisa said, "More than anything, I wish donor sperm could be an option for us. It isn't an option for Bill. There is a part of me that resents his feelings about donor sperm. I resent that he will not even consider it, at least at this point, but I also understand and respect his rights to his feelings."

➤ Accept that grief is a necessary part of the infertility experience. Many people do not understand that grief plays an important role in acceptance and healing. It is vital that you understand you have every right to grieve the loss of your fertility. Also know that the ways people grieve vary, and it is important to let your spouse grieve as he or she chooses.

Elaine and Monte dealt with their pain so differently that they were unable to comfort each other at all. Monte said, "Elaine grieved very openly, with lots of tears and emotional tirades. She wanted me to do the same, and when I didn't, Elaine felt that I didn't care. But I couldn't dredge up all that misery all the time. Open grieving made me feel that our situation was hopeless, but one way I found to grieve without anyone knowing was by taking off and riding roller coasters all day. There were days that I went to the amusement park and forced all of the grief and pain I had inside of me out with my screams."

➤ Understand that you will experience a wide gamut of emotions in your quest to have a child. Many of the people interviewed for this book said they did not seek outside help because they felt that their feelings were abnormal. They felt ostracized enough from society without admitting all of the emotions that had been evoked by infertility. Feelings of jealousy, anger, hate, sadness, self-repulsion, and depression are very common when you are infertile. It is important for the infertile individual to realize that these and other emotions are not abnormal. And if depression leads to serious consideration of suicide, it is vital to get professional help.

Lois experienced long stretches of depression and hopelessness, followed by a brief glimpse of hope when she thought she might be pregnant. When she realized she wasn't, she gave in to anger—at herself, her husband, her doctor, at God, at everything. She said, "I remember thinking I was pregnant the night before my period started. The next morning I skipped into the bathroom, ready to take a home pregnancy test. I pulled down my underwear and saw that it was saturated with blood. I couldn't believe it. I was furious, and I started demolishing the bathroom. I pulled down the curtains, I knocked the shelving down, and I scrawled four-letter words on the mirror with my lipstick. After the rage started to dissipate, I sat in the middle of the mess I had made. My husband came home a little later and asked me if it had been truly necessary to trash the room. I smiled at him and said, 'Yes, it was. Thanks for asking.' For me, it was better to act on my rage than to swallow it and let it eat at my soul."

➻ Refuse to let others tell you how to feel. Well-meaning friends and family may tell you that you are not being rational. They may give you advice on the "appropriate" way to feel. Let them know, in no uncertain terms, that even though they may think your feelings are inappropriate, they are your feelings. Make sure, though, that if your feelings are directed at a person, not to act on them in a destructive or hostile way.

My experiences with friends and co-workers during infertility wasn't always positive, and I haven't been able to 'forgive and forget' everything that happened. Infertility was my constant companion for four years before I got pregnant. Mary, my daughter, is wonderful—everything I ever dreamed of. But I can't stop thinking about how resentful I still am towards one of my co-workers. She knew of my trials with infertility, but before I was even pregnant, she asked me to explain to her the maternity coverage our employer offered. She knew I had researched the coverage thoroughly for my own knowledge. As painful as it was for me, I did as she asked, and three months later she announced her pregnancy.

Even though I have Mary, I still feel rage towards her. My husband told me I should not be petty, and that I should feel happy for her. I couldn't at the time, and I won't feel guilty for it, either.

➻ Put feelings of guilt in perspective. The infertile person's life can be filled with guilt: guilt for having a body that refuses to produce a child, guilt for resenting others who are pregnant, guilt for not wanting to socialize with friends and family, guilt for feeling depressed, guilt for testing the marital relationship, guilt for wanting a baby, guilt for not wanting to accept options other than trying to have a biological child, and guilt for hoping that others will help you. And these are just the tip of the iceberg. You cannot constantly feel guilty for everything, because if you do, you will not survive infertility—you will be too busy berating yourself.

Jean, a woman I've had several discussions with at support group meetings, told me, "When the low-tech treatments did not help us get pregnant, we looked at in vitro fertilization as an option. I remember thinking I would like to try it, but I kept having these nagging doubts. As I talked to my support group, however, I realized that the doubts were really feelings of guilt. We already had a son, and my husband's parents constantly worried about how much money we were spending to have another. They kept insinuating that we were depriving our son. One cycle of IVF was ten thousand dollars, and although we had the money, I kept thinking of my in-laws' comments and feeling such guilt for even considering it."

➡ Refuse to let infertility rule your life. You cannot let infertility consume your every waking moment. It is important to allow yourself time away from infertility. Don't abandon all of your activities for the sake of pursuing infertility treatments. Putting your entire life on hold will not solve your infertility, and if you choose to do so, you will inadvertently reduce some of your available coping techniques.

Jean found that coping with her infertility meant just walking away from it all for awhile. She said, "After four years of extensive treatments I just said, 'hold it.' We hadn't been on vacation during this entire time. So we used the money for a month's treatment to go to the beach for a week. By doing so we made a conscious decision to put off treatment for a month. My husband and I had a wonderful time getting to know each other again, and we felt a little empowered by our decision. For once, we said 'no' to our infertility instead of our infertility telling us 'no.'"

➡ Empower yourself in any way possible. Infertility is a loss of control, and you need to feel that you have some control over your life. Find ways that help you feel in control of your life. You may find empowerment by researching infertility, writing about your loss, finding an appropriate doctor for yourself, choosing when to pursue treatments, deciding what treatments you will have, or making the choice to discontinue infertility treatments. There are many ways to feel more in control of your life. You need to make a conscious effort to look for these tools of empowerment.

Nicole found strength in learning about the options open to her and her husband, Jason. "Researching infertility treatments and adoption made me feel like I could take control of my life. It helped me focus on something else, even if it was only for a day."

➤ Try not to compare your infertility situation to those of others. Know that everyone has different problems and different coping strategies. Options and decisions that are right for someone else may not be right for you. Your situation is unique.

Lois has found the strength to deal with infertility for many years, but admits it hasn't been easy. "When I first found out that we were infertile I began to become obsessed about the injustice of our situation. After all, there were so many people who could become parents in the blink of an eye and would make lousy parents. I realized at that point that to survive, I could not let myself compare my life to fertile peoples' lives. But then I fell into the trap of comparing my life to other infertile peoples' lives.

"I had gone to a lecture on the emotional impact of infertility. The couple speaking had struggled for three years before they achieved a pregnancy. I found myself thinking that they weren't worthy of a child; after all, I had been trying for seven years and had gone through a lot more hell than they had ever dreamed of. I then realized that I was obsessing again, making up this rating scale of infertility in my head. I knew it wasn't helpful to me, and I forced myself to stop comparing my situation to others. That is the only way you can live with irony and injustice."

➤ Find outlets for your emotions. It is vital to find a way to deal with the emotional whirlpool of infertility. Some people find relief though counselors, support groups, talking with close friends, hobbies, or physical activities. There are many ways to release tension, and you should make it a priority to find a way to deal with the stress infertility causes in your life.

The emotional ups and downs of infertility were very difficult for me and at times I felt very alone. I think one of the main reasons I survived infertility was because I had a good friend who listened to me when I needed to talk. I wasn't emotionally ready to go to a counselor or a support group. By being able to share with her, I got the release I needed without having to blurt out my inadequacies to strangers. I cried, grieved, and told her my innermost feelings. She was always there for me, and the best part was that I never had to apologize for what I said. I named my daughter after her, because she helped me find the strength to continue on with treatments. I don't think she will ever know how grateful I am to her.

➤ As difficult as it may seem at first, you can learn to see the humor in your experiences. Infertility is a condition that is extremely difficult to cope with. It is an emotionally-charged experience, and little is written about its effects. If you let it, infertility will drag you down to its deepest depths, and that is precisely why you need to let go of some of the pain and find the humor in your life whenever possible. When you laugh, you can begin to heal.

I found only five seconds of humor on one of the worst days of my life, but it may have been what got me and my husband through to the next day. I remember sitting on the examining table—the doctor had just left the room. He had just confirmed, after four days of spotting, that I was miscarrying the baby I had worked to conceive for four years. It was a horrible, awful time, but as he left the room I turned to my husband and through my tears mimicked the doctor's 'this is it—live with it' attitude. We both started laughing, and it felt so good. It lasted only a moment, before the pain returned, but it broke a chink in depression's armor. I knew I could deal with this loss in time.

➤ Correct myths about infertility as you hear them being spread. There are many myths that people accept as truth which contribute to insensitive remarks, jokes about procedures, and uneducated judgments about infertility treatments. In order to survive infertility, you cannot stand by as these myths are spread. Educate people about the facts of infertility.

When Kyle and Sara chose to adopt, they were confronted with a popular misconception. Sara said, "As we began to make plans for adoption, it seemed like everybody told us, 'You know that a lot of people get pregnant after they adopt.' I always respond by saying that it happens in only about five percent of all cases—not exactly a lot of people. I think myths like this one have to be stopped so they don't raise false hopes."

➤ Understand that you cannot change the fact of your infertility. If you are in denial, you cannot make the best decisions for yourself. You must accept your infertility to do that. Accepting it does not mean you should discontinue treatments or that you need to accept child-free living, however.

Not long ago in our society, infertility wasn't discussed. It was kept quiet, like some secret shame. I found it difficult to admit, even to myself, that it was a reality. It took me awhile to come to terms with my infertility. I now have a child, and will start treatments again to try and have another. No matter how many children I am able to bear, however, I realize I will die an infertile woman. At first I fought it, but now I think of my infertility as a badge of courage.

➛ Talk with close friends and family members, either as a group or individually, about how you would like them to react to you and your infertility. Do not expect your loved ones to read your mind. The longer you wait to discuss your wishes with them, the more distance there may be between you. If their comments hurt you, discuss it with them. Try and come to an agreement on ways to deal with insensitivities. You will find that you will need these people in your life to support you. Help them to understand your needs before withdrawing from them.

My family didn't know how to react to my infertility, and somehow always managed to say or do the wrong thing. After two and a half years of being hurt by my mother's comments, I finally made my needs clear. I feel so stupid for wasting all that precious time. Instead of confronting her and telling her which remarks hurt me, I had swallowed them. I had found myself drifting further and further apart from her. Then one day I finally let it all hang out, and that was when she finally understood what I needed from her.

WHAT EVERY FERTILE PERSON SHOULD KNOW

All of the people I interviewed asked that a section be included in this book which pertained to fertile people who want to help a friend or family member dealing with infertility. One woman even asked for a list of things a mother could say to comfort an infertile daughter. Unfortunately, there is no magical list of the 'right' sentiments. Every infertile individual is unique, and depending on the person's mood at any given time, he or she might need different demonstrations of support. It is possible, however, to offer some basic guidelines.

IF YOU WOULD LIKE TO HELP A PERSON
SURVIVE INFERTILITY, YOU SHOULD:

➤ Acknowledge their situation and their right to grieve. You may not know the exact words to say, and so decide to say nothing. By doing this, however, you are ignoring the infertile person's loss. Nothing is as painful as silence.

Pete, who recently spoke to our support group, remembered how difficult it was find anyone to talk to about his infertility. "The news of my infertility hit me like a meteor. I went home and stewed over it for hours. I remember calling my brother on the phone and telling him what I had just found out. In a matter of seconds he had changed the subject, and was talking about the scores from the basketball game he was watching. We had always been close, and I wanted him to help me accept the news. But he never said a word about my loss. I hung up the phone even more depressed than when I placed the call."

➤ Listen when the person needs an ear. Realize that an infertile person needs you to acknowledge their pain. They have no need for a pep talk, or for glib advice.

After hearing so many people hastily change the subject or recite the same inaccurate platitudes when confronted with her infertility, Nicole found one person's attitude refreshing. "I had a friend who told me she couldn't imagine being in my shoes, and I found that very comforting. She told me that she had no idea how to talk to me or even what she should feel for me. To me, that was the most open and honest thing anyone ever told me."

➤ Refrain from judging the infertile person's decisions, actions, or reactions. Being infertile means making some very tough decisions. It is an emotionally wrenching experience. Even if their decisions or reactions seem inappropriate to you, remember that you are not in their shoes. You have not felt the desperation and have not experienced the same loss they have.

When she began infertility treatment, Lisa was surprised by her mother's attitude. Lisa said, "Before I took the Clomid, I had talked to my mom about taking it. She said, 'Oh Lisa, I wish you wouldn't do that. I just want you to have one grandbaby. I don't want you to have a whole litter.' It just cut me to the quick."

➤ Avoid prying into an infertile couple's decisions. When they are ready to share information, they will do it. Prying will only make the couple resent you. Let them come to you with information.

I have never made a secret of my infertility, but I was not pleased to find it had become a coffee break topic. I had been very open with some of my friends at work. I felt it helped me cope more effectively. But there were some people I did not want to open up to, and most of them respected that. You can imagine my shock when one woman came up to me and asked if I had tried donor-inseminated cycles yet. I told her it was none of her business, and walked out. I still get angry when I think of her question.

➤ Offer your support verbally, through written notes, or through little pick-me-up gifts. The gesture can mean the world to the infertile person. Notes and gifts are especially good, because they can provide support over and over again.

During our struggle with infertility I often found myself alone in my office, working late, with no one to talk to. It was easy to get depressed at times like that. One thing that helped me through infertility was my collection of notes and letters. My husband and one of my friends would write me inspirational notes when I was really low. I always was so grateful to get them. I kept them in a little box, and when I needed inspiration, I'd drag them out and reread them. I have since put all the notes into my child's baby book so that someday she can see how wonderful her father and godmother were to me.

➤ Research information on infertility so that you can be educated as to what the problem actually is and what treatments it might entail. If you have an idea of what the couple is going through emotionally, physically, and financially, you will be better able to respond to them. Be careful not to use your new knowledge to pass along unsolicited advice, however.

Laura, who has not had problems with infertility, took the time to read about the subject to help her understand a friend's situation. "When one of my friends told me she was considering IVF I started researching the process. I was shocked at the cost and the preparations that went into it. I think I became more awed by her resolve to have a baby than ever before. I don't think I could have gone through everything she has. I admire her strength."

➤ Avoid making jokes about infertility and its consequences. If you refuse to laugh at infertility, you are making a statement to both the infertile couple and society. While it is healthy for an infertile couple to find the humor in their experiences, infertility itself is not a laughing matter.

A woman at a support group meeting couldn't even wait to get her coat off before she was complaining about more misinformation being dispensed in the guise of humor. She said, "I was appalled when I heard about this new movie coming out. It's about a woman who had used donor sperm. The plot-line had a black woman asking for an educated black donor and ending up receiving a donation from a low-life white donor. I don't find the old 'mix-up at the sperm bank' plotline funny—I think it's misleading. This type of ill-informed fluff, far from being harmless, adds yet another myth about infer-tility to our social consciousness."

➥ Finally, don't ever let any of the following statements or questions slip from your mouth:

"Just relax, and you'll get pregnant."

"Don't think about it."

"Are you pregnant yet?"

"Have you considered adoption?

"There are a lot of babies that are readily available."

"Whose fault is it that you can't have kids?"

"You don't want kids—they're more trouble than they're worth."

"I know how you feel."

"It must be God's will."

"It'll all work out, don't worry."

There are many more such statements that are similar, and they all wound very deeply. If you truly want to help, be honest, and *ask* how to help. Each person is different, and will want you to say and do things that meet their needs. If you are fertile, please be aware that there are many of us who would love to be able to say the same thing about ourselves.

RESOURCES

This list cannot be, nor is it meant to be, all-inclusive. Support groups and services may be available in your community; the organizations listed here can help you find them. Additional help may be found in the phone book, or through your doctor or religious institution.

Adopted Child
P.O. Box 9362
Moscow, ID 83843
(208) 883-1794
Monthly newsletter for adoptive parents.

Adoptive Families of America, Inc.
3333 Highway 100 North
Minneapolis, MN 55422
(612) 535-4829
Support, information and education about international and special needs adoption.

American Fertility Society
2140 11th Ave. S. Suite 200
Birmingham, AL 35205
(205) 933-8494
Publications and information on infertility.

A.P.A.A.
Adoptive Parent Association of America
P.O. Box 20726
Riverside, CA 92516

Compassionate Friends, Inc.
900 Jorie Blvd., P.O. Box 3696
Oak Brook, IL 60522-3696
(312) 990-0010
A national organization for parents who have lost a child.

The Endometriosis Association
8585 N. 76th Place
Milwaukee, WI 53223
(414) 355-2200 or (800) 992-3636
Offers a wide variety of information and support for women with endometriosis.

F.A.C.E.—Families Adopting Children Everywhere
P.O. Box 28058
Baltimore, MD 21239

Ferre Institute, Inc
258 Genesee St. Suite 302
Utica, NY 13502
(315) 724-4348
Brochures, newsletters and other infertility information.

National Committee for Adoption, Inc. (N.C.F.A.)
1933 17th St. N.W.
Washington, DC 20009-6207
(202) 328-1200;
Hotline: (202) 463-7563
Hotline may be used for information and referrals.

N.I.N.E.
National Infertility
Network Exchange
P.O. Box 204
East Meadow, NY 11554

North American Council on Adoptable Children (N.A.C.A.C.)
1821 University Ave. Suite N498
St. Paul, MN 55104
(612) 644-3036
Offers conferences, newsletters, and general information about adoption.

O.P.T.S.—The Organization of Parents Through Surrogacy
National Headquarters
750 North Fairview St.
Burbank, CA 91505
(818) 848-3761

Pregnancy and Infant Loss Center
1421 E. Wayzata Blvd.
Wayzata, MN 55391
(612) 473-9372
National organization providing information, support and referrals.

Resolve, Inc.
1310 Broadway
Somerville, MA 02144
(617) 623-0744
Publishes a quarterly newsletter, offers educational materials, books, emotional support, and referrals, with fifty local chapters across the U.S.

Serono Symposia, U.S.A.
100 Longwater Circle
Norwell, MA 02061
(617) 982-9000 or
(800) 283-8088;
Hotline: (800) 326-3151
Cosponsors infertility symposia across the country. Hotline assists with assessing insurance coverage for fertility treatment.

Share
St. Joseph's Health Center
300 First Capitol Drive
St. Charles, MO 63301
(314) 947-5000
Support for pregnancy loss

Welcome House: Social Services of the Pearl S. Buck Foundation
P.O. Box 181
Green Hills Farm
Perkasie, PA 18944
(215) 249-0100
Information and support for adoption.

ABOUT THE AUTHOR

As detailed in the first chapter of this book, *Infertility: The Emotional Journey* grew out of **Michelle Fryer Hanson**'s personal experience. At the time when her need was greatest, she could not find any books which dealt with the personal side of infertility in sufficient depth. As a result, she decided to write one herself which would help others who are in the midst of emotional pain.

Ms. Hanson has been an instructor in the Human Development Department at South Dakota State University for the past seven years. She lives with her husband and daughter in Brookings, South Dakota. This is her first book.